YOGA
FOR THE
MIND

YOGA FOR THE MIND

A Treatise on Mental
and Philosophical Yoga
by a Western Yogi

Yogi William Zorn

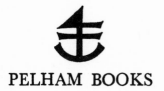

PELHAM BOOKS

First published in Great Britain by
PELHAM BOOKS LTD
52 Bedford Square
*London, W.C.*1
MARCH 1970
SECOND IMPRESSION SEPTEMBER 1972
THIRD IMPRESSION JUNE 1976

ISBN 0 7207 0329 8

Printed in Great Britain by
Hollen Street Press Ltd at Slough
and bound by James Burn at Esher, Surrey

THIS BOOK IS LOVINGLY DEDICATED
TO ALL SINCERE STUDENTS

ACKNOWLEDGEMENTS

I am most grateful to Ruth Mackinnon for reading the manuscript and making many valuable suggestions, thus enabling me to present these sublime teachings more clearly.

This book could not have been attempted but for the dedication and scholarship of the many teachers and writers who have gone before me.

I shall forever be indebted to the great sages whose inspired words are contained within these pages.

W. Z.

CONTENTS

CHAPTER ONE

On Yoga
For The Mind

INTRODUCTION

The mind of man has been the subject of probing study for many centuries. Throughout the ages various views have been expounded regarding the existence, relationships, and true nature of the mind. There are many wonders and mysteries in the universe, but of all these, perhaps none is as wondrous and none more mysterious than the human mind.

The time has passed when Yoga was regarded in the West as something practised only by Indian fakirs who seemed to delight in walking on red-hot coals, drinking poison, and reclining on beds of nails. This mistaken notion gradually has been overcome through an increased flow of objective yogic literature, and through the dedicated efforts of those who themselves had derived great benefits from the practice of Yoga and were anxious for others to share their good fortune.

The aspect of Yoga that enjoys most popularity in the West is the science of Hatha Yoga – that branch of Yoga that deals with the physical body. The spectacular postures that some of the more advanced exponents are able to perform cannot but attract attention. It was soon discovered by those who tried the techniques of Hatha Yoga that an improvement in health rapidly followed. What is not so widely known at present is that Yoga is more than just an unorthodox system for obtaining health.

In a society where so much importance is attached to youthfulness and its accompanying good looks, and where the making of money is often seen as one of the most praiseworthy pursuits,

11

it was perhaps inevitable that in many instances Yoga should become commercialized. Indeed, Yoga has at times been presented to the public as merely a means of obtaining the body beautiful, with the result that serious-minded people turned their backs on Yoga as something without depth. These people may be surprised to learn that Yoga also includes a complete programme of mental training, and that it rests on the world's oldest and most sublime philosophy.

Hatha Yoga is only the beginning of Yoga. The Yoga of the body is but a paving of the way for the Yoga of the mind. The majority of Western people are inclined to believe, especially in light of the upsurging popularity of psychology, that they are the sole authorities on the human mind. However, thousands of years ago, Indian ascetics had already carefully explored man's inner nature. Their findings are today of incalculable value to those who are willing to become acquainted with their teachings, and who are prepared to put them into practice. Here, at once, we strike a vital difference between Western psychology and philosophy on the one hand and Indian psychology and philosophy on the other. The first may be discussed from an armchair, while the latter must be practised and *lived* in order to be fully comprehended.

At first it may seem surprising that techniques that were evolved so long ago are still valid in today's age of scientific discoveries and 'modern' men and women. Yet on closer inspection it will be found that it is not so strange at all. We are still, as were our forefathers, human beings. We are still, as were those who populated this earth before us, wondering what life is all about, and what we really are.

THE YOGIC TEACHINGS

For some this is the best of possible worlds. Busily and happily occupied in the realm of the senses, they have no time for reflection and inner search. For others, however, the wisdom of our ways is open to question. Some turn to religion, finding peace of mind and happiness in the joyful worship of their God. Others seek answers to their burning questions in the study of philosophy. But to many religion and Western philosophy are found wanting, for in this age of science, religious dogmas seem to give birth to as many problems as they solve, while Western philosophy does not offer an entirely satisfactory explanation of the phenomenon of life. Modern man, in his endeavour to overcome a deep sense of insecurity, and discover or retain his own identity, is in dire need of a philosophy that can accommodate the findings of science and that can also answer his questions and misgivings about his own nature.

Today, just as he did in times past, man requires a philosophy for living. Yoga has always been such a philosophy. Its ancient teachings can blend perfectly with present-day ideas and ways of life. Their application gives the practitioner knowledge and security, and prepares him for all eventualities. He becomes so independently strong that even the threat of nuclear holocaust fails to frighten him.

Yoga, in its highest aspects, provides man with definite techniques for knowing and mastering his own mind, as well as a monistic philosophy to reflect upon. As a result of this mental training and philosophical reflection, man can become aware of the essence of his being. In the process he will increase both his willpower and mental strength. He will overcome his fears and gain confidence. He will learn to concentrate. He will establish complete mastery over his thoughts, and will awaken the potentialities that have lain dormant in his mind. Besides all this, he will develop a more profound appreciation of life, and find a new rapport with his fellow man.

Yoga can be practised anywhere. One certainly does not have to set out for the Himalayas and become a hermit, any more than one would have to go to the Holy Land in order to practise Christianity. Yoga teaches us that truth is within us. No matter where one travels, one must still look and seek within. The mind can be trained in any place. The sublime yogic philosophy can be pondered at any time.

The ancient teachings were left to us by the grace of the Indian ascetics. These sages found understanding and happiness for themselves by giving up the life of the world, withdrawing to the forests, and looking deeply into their own minds. Having found the key to wisdom within the depths of their own souls, they devised effective techniques to be followed, which would enable others to make the same exalted discoveries. Their instruction may be followed by anyone who cares to do so. The yogic disciplines as set forth by the ancient masters must be undertaken voluntarily. No one may be told that he *must* do this or that, nor is anyone asked to accept something that goes against his beliefs or his ingrained convictions. The Indian sages were not trying to force their ideas upon anyone. 'Here is the way,' they said. 'Follow this path if you are intent on discovering what you are.'

There is something in Yoga for everyone. Some people will want to conform to its teachings as closely as circumstances allow, without really changing their modes of life. There will be those who discover in their reading exactly what they have been seeking all their lives. There may even be a few who find that what they encounter here, expressed in the words of ancient Indian wisdom, is something they have already attained.

Men and women of all ages and of all races and creeds can benefit from Yoga. The yogic principles are similar in many respects to the Christian ideals, which have exerted such a significant influence on our Western society. Much of Yoga, therefore, can be easily understood and readily accepted by most Occidentals.

Besides what it offers the individual disciple, Yoga provides an ethical code of behaviour which, if accepted universally, would help to make the entire world a better place.

THE MYSTERY OF MAN

Science supplies us with an enormous amount of data about the universe. Looking up at the heavens with our newly acquired knowledge, we may well be excused for falling silent in awe. The universe appears to stretch out infinitely; yet infinite time and distance are incomprehensible to us. During moments like these, man is inclined to regard himself as of little consequence. We are equally awed by the infinitely small atom. But man, caught as he seems to be between the macrocosm and the microcosm, has a body ingeniously built of countless tiny units. He is endowed with feeling, thought, and reason. He himself is one of the universe's greatest wonders.

What is it that holds man together? What is he? In search of answers men turn to religion and philosophy. Some persons find in religion an explanation for all questions; others, more sceptical, bluntly reject religious dogmas. Can we arrive through philosophy at a solution to the mystery that is man? Can critical inquiry lead to understanding? Is reason infallible? Can we ultimately know our real nature? Can we know anything?

The subject of epistemology, or the theory of knowledge, has occupied philosophical minds for thousands of years. As early as 500 B.C., the Sophists doubted that one could really know anything. Consequently, they advanced a doctrine of worldly success, and taught their students the art of influencing people. Since then, from the idealist Plato (427–347 B.C.) to the sceptic Hume (1711–1776) and onward to our own day, the questioning minds of many philosophers have pondered the subject. Plato held that we cannot acquire knowledge through learning, and that all knowledge of forms and universals is already in the mind. Others thought that man only learned from contact with his environment. No sooner would one thinker put forth a plausible concept, than someone else would emerge with a critique and substitute hypothesis. With what one might consider monotonous regularity, theories were postulated and just as quickly refuted. Will this question ever be satisfactorily answered?

The great problems of life were pondered also by the Indian philosophers. Long ago they arrived at answers that they felt fully explained the very essence of being. What is more, they devised methods and techniques through the practice of which subsequent seekers of self-knowledge could also attain their goals.

Can these ancient, foreign teachings be applied successfully in the West, where we live under such different circumstances and are used to such different modes of thinking? It has been said that East and West shall never meet. Is such a contention true, or is it perhaps a fallacy? It certainly is not true from the Eastern viewpoint, for where the West sees diversity and conflict, the East recognizes the possibility of unity. That the teachings of the East can be applied here, today, has been proven by the many men and women now living in America and Europe who have attained through Yoga true and lasting wisdom and happiness.

Socrates said that man's first duty is to heed the injunction 'Know thyself'. On trial for his life in 399 B.C., he maintained that the unexamined life was not worth living. These pronouncements reach across the bridge of time. They are still of the utmost importance today when man seems to be dwarfed by his own scientific inventions, and risks being reduced to a mere number in a computerized world. His frantic efforts to make an impression on his physical environment threaten man with the danger of losing his most precious possession – his own identity. We might well ask what is the good of spectacular scientific progress, if at heart we remain insecure? 'What shall it profit a man if he gain the whole world, and lose his own soul?'

WHAT ARE WE?

René Descartes (1596–1650), the renowned French mathematician and philosopher, lived in an age marked by continuous and severe conflict between religious dogmas on the one hand, and newly emerging philosophical concepts on the other. Fresh ideas began to challenge old and firmly established beliefs. Many people began to question their convictions, and to become sceptical about traditional thought. In this atmosphere of confusion and doubt Descartes sought something that was certain, a concept that would be unshakable in the face of either old or new arguments. Leaving Paris, he retreated to Holland, where he began to reconsider everything he knew, in order to find out if there was anything left that he could still fully accept as reliable knowledge.

Descartes soon discovered that many of his former convictions were built on false beliefs which he had nurtured since his youth. Courageously, he decided to banish from his mind whatever he had any reason to doubt, only to learn that this included just about everything he knew. Finally he arrived at the one fact that he could regard as an absolute certainty – the fact of his own existence. To express this one fundamental certainty, he formulated the now famous dictum *'Cogito, ergo sum'* ('I think, therefore I am'). To Descartes the truth of his proposition was clear every time he uttered it or reflected upon it. For a thought to exist, he reasoned, there must be a thinker.

Whether they agree or disagree with Descartes' celebrated proposition, most men would have little doubt about the fact of their own existence. We feel and know for certain that we *are*. It is the question of *what* we are that has raised such great problems.

Some materialists have tried to explain away man as solely a system of organic matter, conditioned by environment, and subject to the laws of biological process. Surely such a narrow view does not give us the whole picture of the human phenomenon. What if we looked at an apple tree in winter and subsequently defined the tree as a barren object, nothing more? Such a dry and superficial report would account for neither the sweetly fragrant, magnificent blossoms the tree will be covered with in spring, nor for the healthy, delicious fruit it will bear – all surely important factors in any explanation of an apple tree. The materialistic view of man is, thus, a highly unsatisfactory one. It makes man appear a creature devoid of soul, of free will – really nothing more than a piece of machinery. Such an unimaginative depiction does not do man full justice. Where do we fit in his indisputable sense of his own existence? How does the mechanistic picture explain his capacity for introspective reflection? How does it account for the depth of his feelings, the intensity of his emotions? Where does it find the origin of his noble thoughts, high ideals, lofty aspirations, his capacity for selfless action and sacrificial love, his ability to be deeply moved by beauty and nature and to express all these feelings through art?

If we were to hear someone at our door and were to call out, 'Who is there?' the caller would be likely to answer, 'It is I!' adding, perhaps, as clarification, 'You know, Jones!' During the course of only one day, depending on the circumstances, that same person might sincerely declare himself to be: the father of Ruth . . . an American . . . a Freemason . . . the brother of Sonja . . . a Republican . . . a businessman . . . a Texan . . . a philosopher. In his daydreams, or at night when asleep and dreaming vividly, this person might clearly see himself as: a successful general . . . a cool racing-driver . . . a supersalesman . . . a smooth seducer of countless females . . . a statesman changing the course of history. His dream experiences will be as real to him at this time as are his feelings about himself during his waking hours.

If such a person sat down quietly and asked himself which of all these labels characterized his real identity, he would have to admit that none of them accurately, or even adequately, described it; that they all represented only partial, superficial aspects. He would feel that behind all these bits and pieces was something more lasting, something more real. It is through the practice of Yoga that man can find out what this more significant part of his being is.

YOGA FOR THE MIND

This book deals with two branches of Yoga – Raja Yoga and Jnana Yoga. They are to be studied and practised in conjunction, one supplementing the other.

Raja Yoga, or Royal Yoga, is the science of mind control. Through the practice of its techniques the student learns to conquer his mind; once he has finally achieved absolute control, he can experience – in deep meditation – that spark of Infinity within himself that is his real self. *Jnana* means spiritual knowledge, and it is with this that Jnanan Yoga, or the Yoga of Knowledge, deals.

That man does have an eternal principle within his being – whether one calls that principle 'self', 'soul', 'psyche', 'spirit', 'purusha', or 'atman' – is the contention of the Indian sages. It was through prolonged introspection that they made contact with this infinite self. The methods they used are the mind-stilling techniques of Yoga. The sole criterion by which to judge the validity of their teachings is personal experience : the 'proof' that the self exists and can be reached lies in each individual's discovery of his own self. *Yoga* is the Sanskrit term for union. It is derived from the root-verb *yuj*, which means 'to yoke', 'to join'. The various branches of Yoga are but different avenues of approach to the same goal – integration with Infinity. In Raja Yoga the mind is joined to the self; in Jnana Yoga this self, which so far has been regarded as belonging to man, or vice versa, is joined to *Brahman,* the World Soul. Whereas Jnana Yoga inquires into the nature of the universe and of the human soul, which it finds to be identical, in Raja Yoga the self is sought and experienced directly by means of intellect-transcending meditation. In Raja Yoga the instrument used is the will, and in Jnana Yoga the tool is the intellect. This does not mean, however, that Jnana Yoga is a purely intellectual approach. The sages knew that intellect has its limitations, that although it takes the thinker far, it cannot take him all the way. In the end, it is the stilled mind that can fully comprehend. Some people will feel more attracted at first to the practice of mental discipline, preferring to trust intuition rather than intellect. Others revere their thinking powers, and feel irresistibly drawn to the study of Yoga philosophy. One may follow one's inclination in the early stages of training, but all soon find that in order to achieve success in either Raja Yoga or Jnana Yoga, both subjects need to be practised and studied simultaneously.

TO THE STUDENT

If you decide to take up the study and practice of Yoga, you will find it a turning point in your life. There is much to be gained. You must approach the subject positively. The man who has faith succeeds. At first, you may not fully comprehend the magnificence of the ultimate goal – you *cannot* yet appreciate it fully. But as you progress, you will become increasingly aware of it. Although its final attainment may seem distant to you at this stage, remember that all long journeys commence with the first step. Therefore begin at the beginning.

In many of the ancient scriptures, the student is advised to find a personal teacher, a *guru*. This is now no longer necessary. Because there were very few books, and few people were able to read, the sacred teachings were handed down orally for many centuries; and were put down in writing only after perhaps a thousand years. Today, when so many books containing the classics are easily available, the need for a personal teacher is eliminated. The writen word is the best of all *gurus*. Through books the great masters speak to us directly.

The mental training involved in Yoga will result in a change of personality. Consider, therefore, the effect this may have on people close to you. The Yoga student should live in harmony with his surroundings and with other people. He should avoid disturbing others.

There is no set required length of time for practice. To some, success will come only after long striving, while for others realization may come sooner, in a magnificent, all-encompassing flash. Much depends on one's previous mode of life; some come better prepared than others.

The path you are about to follow was laid out meticulously by the masters of yore especially for you and for those like you. Since ancient times, thousands upon thousands have travelled the path. Many thousands are making their way along it on this very day, and countless thousands will proceed along the same route in the future. As you travel, all these seekers are with you in spirit.

The quest for Yoga can be seen as the climbing of a mountain that reaches into the heavens. A path to the top has been hewn out by the great sages, who left guideposts along the way. Standing in the valley, the prospective climber looks up with longing and admiration at the high peak, glistening white against the blue sky. Joyfully, he commences the ascent. Soon, he may discover that there are many obstacles to be overcome. Often the path is steep and strewn with rocks. But no matter how the traveller is equipped, and how difficult he may think the climb, he will derive great assistance from the directions left him by those who went before. If only he perseveres, he will, thanks to their help, finally reach the top. During the journeys, he may become tired, and want to sit down to rest. There are many vantage points where he can relax for a time and view the distance already travelled. This will give him new strength and confidence. Refreshed and intent, he will rise to his feet again and head once more toward his goal, approaching nearer to it with every step.

In the rarefied atmosphere at the summit, he will breathe deeply of the pure air. From the heights, he will view the panorama spread out beneath him as one who has conquered all.

He who has attained Yoga has received the greatest of all gifts: he will possess profound spiritual knowledge, and he will have cast aside the erroneous notion that he is a lone, finite entity. He will have discovered what he really is – infinite, absolute Being.

CHAPTER TWO

The Yoga Sutras
of Patanjali

Exactly when Patanjali lived is not known, but it is generally assumed to have been about 300 or 200 B.C. Our present-day knowledge of dates regarding events and personalities in early Indian history is still quite vague.

Three books are attributed to Patanjali. One is a work on grammar, entitled *Patanjala Bhashya*. Another is *Charaka*, a work on medicine. Finally there are his *Yoga Sutras*, or *Yoga Aphorisms*, which form the textbook of Raja Yoga. The *Yoga Sutras* are regarded as the highest authority on the subject, and are among the most important classical texts of yogic literature. In a series of extremely condensed aphorisms, nearly two hundred in all, divided into four chapters, Patanjali explores the human mind, and lays down strict rules for its control. However, the aphorisms, or *sutras*, do not make easy reading. It must be realized that, besides being a very ancient work, written in a language containing many words for which there are no exact English equivalents, the *Yoga Sutras* are not directed toward beginners, but rather toward those already familiar with Yoga.

Patanjali's main subject is the technique of mind control to be practised by *sadhakas,* or aspirants, intent on self-realization; but his teachings in this respect are surrounded by a mass of religious, metaphysical, and occult speculations. In the present book those aphorisms have been selected and ordered which are of most direct concern to the student interested in actual practice. Technical complications and extraneous issues have been avoided, and each *sutra* has been translated into modern phraseology. In this presentation the student will find a straightforward, workable programme leading to the enjoyment of perfect control and, ultimately, to the attainment of the superconscious state of *samadhi*.

It is entirely up to the individual student to determine how far he wants to proceed with his mental training. The science of Raja Yoga provides a long-range programme which cannot be accomplished in a hurry. The student would be wise to try to master the simpler techniques before he concerns himself with the more advanced methods. As he advances in Yoga, his mind will unfold, and he will be able to do more and to understand more than he had previously thought possible.

For the purposes of exploration and subjugation of the mind, the student should try to regard it as just another organ – to think of it as a sixth sense, as it were. He should tell himself that his mind is subject to him, that by means of his will he can make it obey his commands. In time, he will be able to exercise complete dominance and will hold his mind as 'the charioteer holds his restive horses'.

Even early in his training, the practitioner of mental Yoga will reap worthwhile benefits. In daily life, his mind will function with increased efficiency. Practice of the various mental techniques will lead to a complete relaxation of nervous tension and to the promotion of emotional stability. Nor will the benefits be restricted only to the mind, for the condition of the nervous system has a great influence upon the physical body as well.

Yoga may change the student, but it can only do so for the better, since it lays the foundations of a true and lasting personality.

THE YOGA SUTRAS OF PATANJALI

I, 1 *Now follows an exposition of Yoga.*

The first *sutra* is merely an introduction. In his next *sutra* Patanjali will give a definition of the Yoga he is going to explain.

I, 2 *Yoga is the science of controlling the activities of the mind.*

It is made clear that the form of Yoga about to be taught is Raja Yoga, the science of mind-control. Patanjali's treatise is, in essence, not a philosophical one.

Mind control is considered to be achieved when the mind can be held at will in a state of complete restraint, or *nirodha*. Master of one's thoughts and feelings, one should be able to suspend all conscious mental activities at any given moment, and for any chosen duration of time.

I, 3 *He whose mind is completely still becomes aware of his true nature.*

In this *sutra* Patanjali indicates both the purpose of Raja Yoga, and the way the goal can be achieved. Raja Yoga is practised in order to discover and experience one's essential nature. The technique to be used is that of mental stillness. The following *sutras* explain how absolute tranquillity of the mind can be realized.

Normally, the mind is busily occupied registering the constant stream of messages from the senses, observing the manifold happenings in the immediate surroundings, and thinking various thoughts. A mind thus active is not in a condition to become aware of what lies beyond itself. Only on cessation of all mental functions can the spirit, which, as Yoga teaches, is inherent in man, shine through. This will happen in the last stage of yogic training, when the superconscious state of *samadhi* has been reached.

In an often-quoted analogy, the mind is compared to a lake, and the thoughts in the mind to the waves on the lake. When the water is in turmoil, one cannot possibly see the bottom of the lake. Only when the water is perfectly still does it become crystal clear, and only then can the bottom of the lake be seen. So it is with the mind. As one cannot see through turbulent water, so a mind clouded with thoughts is not conducive to seeing that which is beyond thought. When the mind has stilled completely, man can become aware of what he really is.

I, 4 *As long as the mind is active, man identifies himself with his mind.*

When man is swayed by his feelings and emotions, he sees these feelings and emotions as very real. To him, they represent his essential nature. Only when all mental activities are successfully subdued does he become free from the web of the senses, and only then can he penetrate beyond the mind.

I, 12 *Mental control is brought about by* abhyasa *and* vairagya.

Abhyasa means practice and *vairagya* is the Sanskrit term for nonattachment. As stated, both *abhyasa* and *vairagya* are necessary to achieve control over the mind. They are interdependent; one needs to adopt both methods in order to attain the goal. *Abhyasa* and *vairagya* are more closely defined in subsequent *sutras*.

I, 13 Abhyasa *is the persistent effort to restrain the different mental activities.*

One of the conditions necessary to achieve control over the mind is that one should consistently try to restrain thoughts and emotions. To what extent one should try is emphasized in the next *sutra*.

I, 14 *After a long, uninterrupted struggle,* abhyasa, *applied earnestly and devotedly, will become an established habit.*

Controlling the mind is a task of great magnitude, beside which the achieving of material wealth or worldly fame is child's play. The mind can only be brought under control after a long and hard battle. It is not sufficient to practise just for a short period each day. One should try to control thoughts at every opportunity. If one lets up, hard-won ground will quickly be lost. The struggle should be uninterrupted. One may try now and then, and perhaps even achieve some measure of success, but worthwhile results, at least from a yogic point of view, are obtained only with a hundred per cent effort. If one keeps on trying, earnestly and devotedly, the practice of controlling the thoughts will gradually become a way of life.

I, 15 Vairagya *is the state in which the craving for objects has been overcome.*

The second necessity for victory in the battle for mind control is *vairagya,* or nonattachment. Try as one may, it is useless to attempt to become absolute master over the mind if one does not also try to overcome the desire for worldly objects. As long as there is a craving for power, wealth, and luxury, one will remain a slave of one's desires. These desires must be eliminated.

Western man is often encouraged to believe that in order to be happy, he must be rich. Those who have amassed fortunes, no matter by what means, are likely to be held up to him as shining examples. Many are the stories told to Western man about the advantages of having possessions and wealth. The yogi does not condemn wealth in itself, but only the desire for it.

Although he may, the student of Raja Yogi is not obliged to give away all his possessions, don a yellow robe, and henceforth rely on Providence or on the charity of his fellow men. The Western student may outwardly continue to live his normal life while attempting to practise the inward renunciation which is the only true *vairagya,* and is not achieved by physical renunciation nor impeded by lack of such renunciation.

I, 16 *Absolute* vairagya *comes from awareness of the self.*

In the final stage of Yoga, in *samadhi,* man experiences his true ego – the indwelling spirit that is called the self. This experience has such a powerful effect on the mind that all other impressions, thoughts, and desires are disintegrated. Selfish desires are forever rendered inactive, and nonattachment in its highest form is permanently established.

As long as there has been no self-realization, the seeds of attachment, with all their disturbing characteristics, will remain.

1, 19 *Some people are born yogis.*

While most people will have to work very hard in order to become yogis, as explained in the next *sutra*, to a few Yoga will come naturally. These are the people who are selfless and content by nature, and who are spiritually attuned to a high degree. Without the need for study, they possess a profound insight into their own nature, the nature of others, and of all that is.

I, 20 *Others attain success in Yoga only through faith, persistent effort, recollection, and the application of a keen intellect.*

There are many different kinds of people, all with different characteristics. As mentioned in the previous *sutra*, some people are born yogis. However, there are also people who have to pass through a lifetime of trial and error before they see the Light. Between these two extremes, there are many variations. Some require more time and effort in order to succeed in Yoga than do others.

Faith—both in the goal and in the methods applied—is needed in order to attain the highest.

Without persistent effort, there will be no worthwhile result.

The student should be able to remember his past deeds, and to recollect their consequences, so as to learn from his mistakes.

Intellectually-minded people will want to reason as far as their intellects can take them. They should study Yoga philosophy as well as making a persistent effort to control their minds.

I, 21 *Success in Yoga comes most quickly to those who desire it most strongly.*

The more intense one's longing to succeed, the sooner will one accomplish one's intention. This is true in almost any endeavour.

I, 22 *The measure of success in Yoga depends on whether one tries little, moderately, or intensely.*

The Yoga student is not threatened with damnation if he does not try very hard. He is simply held to be wanting in desire for yogic progress, and he is thought of as not being ready for the advanced teachings. The rules to be followed are laid down as guidelines by the ancient sages, and it is up to the student to make use of them. If his efforts are only half-hearted, he will remain bogged down in the play of nature, and in spiritual ignorance.

I, 30 *Disease, laxity, doubt, carelessness, laziness, worldliness, wrong views, lack of success, and instability are obstacles that distract the mind.*

Many are the distractions that come to man. All are obstacles that have to be overcome.

If the body is not healthy, it will distract the mind and concentration will be extremely difficult. It is for this reason that Hatha Yoga, or physical Yoga, is regarded as an essential preliminary to Raja Yoga. *Mens sana in corpore sano* (a sound mind in a sound body).

A man who is lax is unlikely to succeed.

When there is doubt about the validity of the teachings, any attempt to follow them can only be half-hearted.

A casual aproach to Yoga will almost certainly bring very little or no result.

Mental apathy is a great drawback.

If the worldly life holds too many attractions, Yoga practice will suffer accordingly.

If the student has a mistaken notion about the true purpose of Yoga, he will remain lost in the wilderness of the senses.

Failure to attain a stage of Yoga, or failure to establish oneself securely in that stage, can only be blamed on a lack of zeal or consistency.

I, 31 *Grief, despair, lack of control over the body, and irregular breathing are the symptoms of an uncontrolled mind.*

These symptoms will disappear as the student progresses with his Yoga training.

I, 32 *For the removal of obstacles, there should be constant practice of one principle.*

The student should constantly bear the yogic ideals in mind, and try to conform to the yogic teachings as best he can. Many people disperse their energies by hopping from one system, or philosophy, to another, but for one who is intent on speedy success in Yoga this is a useless technique. He should polarize his efforts, and practise Yoga to the (temporary) exclusion of everything else.

I, 33 *The mind becomes calm by adopting a mental attitude of friendliness toward happiness, of compassion toward misery, of gladness toward good, and of indifference toward evil.*

The subject under discussion in this *sutra* is how to achieve calmness of mind. The student's main interest at this stage is to achieve or maintain his mental equilibrium. By feeling either elated or depressed about something that happens in the outside world, or in regard to something that is done to him, he creates a mental disturbance. Life with its pleasurable and painful interludes goes on, and the student should not become too deeply involved in all this, at least not at his present stage. He will first have to change himself before he can set out to change the world.

I, 34 *Calmness of mind is also promoted by the practice of breathing exercises.*

The science of Yoga includes specific breathing techniques which are practised to bring about mental equilibrium. These are called *pranayama,* or *pranayama* exercises. They are fully discussed in Chapter IV of this book.

I, 35 *The increasing strength of the mental faculties helps to make the mind steady.*

When the student brings his studies into practice, the resulting development of mental power will be of great help to him in calming his mind. The stronger he becomes, the less outside happenings will influence him. As far as his own mental activity is concerned, he will be able to tell his mind to be calm, and in time it will quickly obey his command.

I, 36 *Serenity of mind also follows awareness of the Inner Light.*

The first glimpse of the self has a profound effect on the mind, and great peace ensues.

I, 37 *The mind becomes calm by thinking of a selfless person.*

If the student knows a person who is not selfish, thoughts about that person will have a peace-inducing effect on his mind. He may hold this particular person as his example, and if he encounters situations in life where he is in doubt as to his correct attitude, he may ask himself how this selfless person would act under the same circumstances.

II, 3 *The causes of misery are* avidya, asmita, raga, dvesa, *and* abhinivesa.

The five causes of misery are called the five *klesas*. Through the practice of Yoga the *klesas* are rendered powerless. Exactly what each *klesa* is will be explained in the following *sutras* and commentaries.

II, 4 Avidya *is the reason for the other causes of misery, be they dormant, hardly noticeable, scattered, or overwhelming.*

Ignorance, or *avidya, is not ignorance of things of the world,* but ignorance in spiritual matters. When man realizes that he is not a small, separate entity lost in the vastness of the universe, but instead is an integral part of the One Life, the pain-bearing obstructions are destroyed.

II, 5 Avidya *is mistaking the limited, the impure, the painful, and the nonself for the eternal, the pure, the good, and the self, respectively.*

When one has a limited or wrong idea about the nature of the self, which is eternal and omnipresent, one is held down by ignorance, or *avidya,* and subject to egotism, attachment, aversion, and the clinging to life.

II, 6 Asmita *is identifying the seer with the instrument of seeing.*

First we think that the eye is the organ of vision, but later we learn that the real seat of vision is in the mind. First we think that the mind is us, later we learn that our real identity is beyond mind.

II, 7 Raga, *or attachment, results from pleasure.*

From the experiencing of pleasure, attachment develops. The pleasurable experience, be it physical, mental, or emotional, causes an impression in the mind, which would like the experience continued or repeated. In this way an attachment is formed.

Raga, or attachment, carries within it the seed of misery. We fear to lose that to which we are attached.

Does the Yoga student have to give up all pleasures? No, he may enjoy pleasure as it comes to him, but he should learn to be able to do without pleasurable experiences. The danger lies not in pleasure itself, but in the attachment to it. The student should attempt to overcome his dependence on, and desire for, sensual gratification. While enjoying pleasure, he should ever be ready to give it up.

II, 8, Dvesa, *or aversion, results from pain.*

We cringe from that which brings us pain. We do not want a painful experience repeated, and so *dvesa,* or aversion, develops. The pain is not necessarily physical, it can also be emotional or mental. We develop *dvesa* just as much from unhappiness as from physical pain.

Raga and *dvesa* are mind-disturbing factors, and therefore the student should overcome them.

II, 9 Abhinivesa, *or the clinging to life, dominates even the learned.*

The will to live is inherent in living things. However, the physical body will not exist forever in its present form. The student should become strong enough and wise enough to accept this fact gracefully. A man who is afraid can never be master over his mind. Fear disturbs the mind.

Through the practice of Raja Yoga, the student learns to remain calm under all circumstances.

II, 11 *The manifestations of the five* klesas *are to be suppressed by meditation.*

Through meditation the five pain-bearing obstructions are to be banished from the mind. One reflects intently on the origin, manifestations, and meaning of the five *klesas*. Once the *klesas* are isolated, and once they are regarded purely as distractions, their disturbing influence will be nullified.

II, 10 *The seeds of the* klesas *can be conquered by dissolving them into their causal state.*

By means of meditation the *klesas* are made inactive, but are not fully destroyed. In time they can come again into the field of consciousness. As long as *avidya,* or spiritual ignorance, exists, the *klesas,* rooted in *avidya,* remain potential dangers. In self-realization *avidya* is dissolved, and with it all the *klesas.*

II, 26 *Unbroken practice of discrimination is the means of destruction of* avidya, *or spiritual ignorance.*

Ignorance in spiritual matters is overcome by the study of the yogic scriptures, and by the continuous contemplation of the meaning and implications of the teachings therein.

II, 28 *By the practice of the different stages of Yoga the impurities in the mind are destroyed, and spiritual knowledge will arise and lead to awareness of Reality.*

Before the eight stages of Yoga are set out in the next *sutra,* the purpose of yogic practice is once more explained. Yoga is practised to calm the mind, so that man can become aware of his true nature and the nature of everything. There are many different yogic techniques, but all have one thing in common – their final aim is to purify the mind so that it becomes a fit instrument for the attainment of spiritual knowledge and supersensuous experience.

II, 29 *The eight steps of Yoga are* yama, niyama, asana, pranayama, pratyahara, dharana, dhyana *and* samadhi.

Yama	– Abstention
Niyama	– Observance
Asana	– Posture
Pranayama	– Breath Control
Pratyahara	– Sense withdrawal
Dharana	– Concentration
Dhyana	– Meditation
Samadhi	– Identification

Raja Yoga, like any science, requires preparation, and follows its own proven method.

Yama and *niyama* are moral disciplines, and they are the first requirements in the student's quest for perfection.

Asana and *pranayama* fall in the field of Hatha Yoga (physical Yoga).

Dharana, dhyana, and *samadhi* form internal Yoga, or mental Yoga, to which *pratyahara* can also be added.

In the following *sutras,* each yogic step in turn is discussed, some in more detail than others.

II, 30 Yamas *are noninjury, continence, nongreed, truthfulness, and nonstealing.*

The five *yamas,* or abstinences, constitute the first rung of the ladder to Yoga. Together with the five *niyamas,* or observances, described in II, 32, they form an ethical code of very high standard to which the student should adhere to the best of his knowledge and ability. It is impossible to achieve any worthwhile and lasting success in Yoga if one knowingly lives in contradiction to the defined abstinences and observances. If they cannot be followed to the letter, one should earnestly attempt to live up to the idea embodied in them.

Noninjury (*ahimsa*). First, and significantly so, is the principle of noninjury. The Yoga student should try to avoid causing harm to man or beast in thought, word, or deed. The infliction of physical or mental pain on others is against the first rule of Yoga. As the student progresses, he will learn to see the oneness of life, and far from wanting to harm, he will develop a deep love for all creatures.

Continence (*bramacharya*). Absolute continence is only possible, or desirable, for a very few people. Those who feel called upon to abstain from sex altogether should do so. Those who are called upon, either by temperament or through circumstance, to perform the sexual act, should attempt to avoid over-indulgence in lustful actions and thoughts. They should try to moderate, in sexual expression, as in everything else. Sex, as every other aspect of life, is a great wonder, and should be appreciated as such. He who performs the sexual deed should act it out with a sense of awe and humility.

Nongreed (*aparigraha*). We must have the necessities of life, but there is a limit. Many people want much more than they need, and often they desire things just for the sake of possessing them. This is what should be overcome. Selfish desires have been, and will be, the cause of much unhappiness in the individual and in the world. The Yoga student should try to rise above the misery-causing characteristic of greed. He can never make his mind calm so long as he entertains selfish thoughts.

Truthfulness and nonstealing are moral virtues whose worth is self-evident.

II, 32 Niyamas *are purity, contentment, austerity, study, and devotion to Divinity.*

Here the five *niyamas,* or observances, are given.

The student should aim for purity – not only purity of body, but, especially, purity of mind. He should try to entertain only pure thoughts.

B

Contentment (*santosha*). A feeling of contentment will be developed if the student focuses his attention on the favours life has bestowed upon him.

Austerity (*tapas*). Not the punishing of the flesh, but the ability to live on the bare necessities of life and to be able to endure hardship is *tapas*. Austerity is an essential way of life for one who is intent not on the riches of the external world, but rather on the immense wealth of the inner life. *Tapas* is not just an outward way of life; if this were so it would be a waste of effort. Living a physically austere life, while dreaming of worldly riches, is not true austerity. *Tapas* should be in the mind more than anywhere else.

The study to be performed is the study of one's own mind, and of the yogic scriptures that deal with the great questions of life and the existence and nature of the self.

Devotion to Divinity. Patanjali's philosophy is a religious one. He calls Divinity *Ishvara*, which he describes as a special soul, untouched by the afflictions of life, actions and the result of actions (I, 24). In Him is infinite wisdom (I, 25). He, being unlimited by time, gave inspiration to the ancient teachers (I, 26). His designation is *Om* (I, 27).

Religious students will readily recognize the deity of their beliefs in what Patanjali terms *Ishvara*, devotion to Whom will result in Illumination (I, 23; II, 45). Yoga can be studied and practised by people of all religious denominations; in fact, in these people it should intensify devotion to their Master.

Nonreligious students may read in the fifth observance a command to develop a sense of awe at the wonder which is Life.

In another part (II, 1) of Patanjali's *Yoga Sutras*, the last three *niyamas* – austerity, study, and devotion to Divinity – are said to constitute Kriya Yoga, which is practised (II, 2) to destroy the pain-bearing obstructions and to bring about *samadhi*, the eighth and highest yogic stage.

II, 33 *To annihilate impure thoughts, contrary thoughts should be pondered.*

Purity, the first of the five observances, is, foremost, mental purity. This *sutra* presents a direct and effective technique to be used for the suppression of thoughts contrary to the high yogic ideals. Evil, destructive, and negative thoughts are purposely replaced by virtuous, constructive, and positive reflections.

Thoughts of hate should be replaced by thoughts of love, sorrow by joy, greed by contentment, dishonesty by uprightness, fear by courage, weakness by willpower, and selfish desires should be eradicated through thoughts of unselfishness.

II, 34 *Impure thoughts and deeds — whether slight, medium or intense; whether committed, caused or abetted; whether through greed, anger, or confusion — result in misery and ignorance. Therefore the method of substituting contrary thoughts is applied.*

If there was any doubt about the undesirability of entertaining thoughts adverse to the yogic ideals, this doubt is here dispelled. Impurity causes misery and ignorance.

II, 41 *From mental purity arises cheerfulness, the ability to concentrate, and control over the senses. Thus the mind will become fit for the realization of the self.*

Once again the importance of the first of the five *niyamas,* purity, is stressed. The establishment of mental purity has far-reaching results, as we see from this *sutra.* Control over the senses is the fifth step of Yoga. Concentration represents the sixth stage. Realization of the self is the goal of Yoga. The groundwork for ultimate success in Yoga is laid by thinking pure thoughts.

II, 38 *By the establishment of continence vigour is gained.*
Patanjali does not moralize on the subject of sex. Instead, he states briefly that the steady practice of *brahmacharya,* or continence, leads to the gaining of energy.

It is obvious that there is an expenditure of physical energy in the performance of the sexual act. Overindulgence reduces physical stamina and depletes the nervous system. Therefore sexual activity should be curtailed. Mental energy is also dissipated by constant thoughts about sex. Mental energy can be redirected into other avenues, and utilized for spiritual purposes.

However, there are people who are constituted in such a way they feel the sexual urge very strongly. For them, the repression of a basic instinct like the sexual impulse would demand too much energy. In the long run they conserve energy, and achieve a more balanced state of mind, by giving in to nature in a limited way.

II, 42 *From contentment comes great happiness.*

Once a state of *santosha,* or contentment, has been cultivated, happiness will follow. Contentment, should become a habit.

People often think that they will be happy once they attain a particular worldly goal they have set themselves. However, they will probably discover on reaching that goal, that they still are not happy. True happiness comes not from outward success, but from within.

The Yoga student should learn to be content with his lot in life. Instead of grumbling, he should fulfil his duties to the best of his abilities, glad to be of service to the community. It does not matter whether his job seems important or trivial. The student will try to progress in the world until he realizes that this is not his true purpose in life. Instead, he should devote his energy to the practice of Yoga. His desire for progress should centre not so much on success in a worldly sense as on the mastering of his own mind.

II, 43 *Perfection of the sense organs and the body is arrived at through destruction of impurities by austerity.*

In this *sutra* the results of the practice of *tapas,* or austerity, are declared. Here the impurities mentioned are physical impurities, the destruction of which is helped along by the living of an austere life. Overindulgence in food and comfort is detrimental to physical and mental health.

II, 46 Asana *is a firm and comfortable posture.*

The third step of Yoga – *asana,* or posture – receives little attention in Patanjali's treatise, yet an essential point is made here. A yogic posture should be firm but at the same time comfortable. Firmness of seat is required so that one remains alert, and comfort in posture is necessary in order not to distract the mind. If there is pain or exaggerated muscular tension, it is very difficult, if not impossible, to focus the mind on things other than the body. See Chapter III of this book for some further details on *asanas.*

II, 49 *When* asana *has been mastered,* pranayama, *which is the control of inhalation, follows.*

The fourth step of Raja Yoga is *pranayama.* The aim of the practice of *pranayama* is to check the velocity of the mind. *Pranayama* is the connecting link between physical and mental Yoga.

For a complete listing of the classical *pranayama* exercises, together with detailed instructions, see Chapter IV of this book.

II, 53 *Through the practice of* pranayama, *the mind becomes fit for* dharana.

Dharana means concentration, which is the sixth step of Yoga. The present *sutra* emphasizes that control over the breath is preliminary to control over the mental faculties.

II, 54 Pratyahara *is the detachment of the senses from the objects of sense.*

The five senses – sight, hearing, touch, taste, and smell – constantly react to the outside world. Their messages come in an uninterrupted flow to the brain. If one were constantly paying attention to this flood of incoming messages, one would have very little time to do anything else. In order to concentrate one must be able to withdraw one's consciousness from the sense organs. The student becomes distracted if, for example, he feels a strain in his legs, if he hears a conversation in another room, if he observes a fly walking on the wall, if he smells food being prepared, or if he can still taste his last meal in his mouth. He must learn to disregard all these distractions, and concentrate on whatever object or subject he has chosen. The mind needs to be isolated from the external world.

Pratyahara can be a natural process. For example, when we are completely absorbed in reading an interesting book, we feel neither heat, cold, nor discomfort, and we may not even hear our name being called, a sound we normally react to very alertly.

When the student is ready for *dharana,* the sixth stage of Yoga, he will be able to concentrate on the internal process of his mind. In that case *pratyahara* follows automatically.

III, 1 Dharana *is the condition in which the mind is confined to one object.*

Dharana, or concentration, is the sixth step of Yoga. Here the student must learn to hold the attention of his mind to one thing or one thought. With *dharana* internal Yoga begins. All the student's previous training has been a preparation for the art of controlling the mind. Bodily and mental disturbances have been reduced to a minimum. By leading a chaste, austere, and unselfish life, tendencies in the student's mind have been subdued to a great extent. His body has become healthy, or has maintained its health, through the practice of physical Yoga. He can sit for prolonged periods. Breath control has calmed his mind, and he has attempted to disregard the messages from the sense. All in all, the student has had a thorough preliminary training. He will need it, because real concentration is difficult. The subject of concentration is fully discussed in Chapter V of this book. This chapter also includes forty mental exercises for the improvement of concentration.

III, 2 Dhyana *is the condition in which uninterrupted attention is paid to the object of concentration.*

The seventh step of Yoga is *dhyana,* or meditation, which is a prolonged and deepened form of concentration. Distractions no longer come into the field of consciousness, interrupting the concentration process. The practitioner can hold his mind on the chosen object for any amount of time he desires. Nevertheless, a duality still exists. While in *dhyana,* the student remains aware, however vaguely, that he is meditating. Once he loses this notion, *dhyana* turns into *samadhi.*

Chapter VII of this book is wholly devoted to the art of meditation.

III, 3 Samadhi *is the condition in which there is only consciousness of the object of meditation, and no awareness of the mind itself.*

The eighth and last step of Yoga is *samadhi,* or identification. *Samadhi* is concentration in the highest degree. There are no distractions, and the mind has shed all notion of its separate existence. It is devoid of its own nature, as it were, and is aware only of the object.

In *samadhi* the meditator is lost in the object of meditation. He identifies himself with it.

According to Patanjali's teaching there are various types of *samadhi;* but in yogic literature as a whole, the unqualified term *samadhi* has been extensively used to denote the state wherein the self is directly experienced. Patanjali, in his *sutra* IV, 29, calls this final state *dharma-megha-samadhi.*

Chapter VIII of this book is devoted to a discussion of the blissful state of *samadhi.*

I, 41 *As pure crystal takes on the colour of its surroundings, so in the mind from which distractions have been expelled, knower, knowing, and known become one.*

The simile used in this *sutra* illustrates what happens during *samadhi.* If we place a crystal on a red surface, the crystal will appear to be red. If it is a flawless gem, it will be, at least to our vision, completely absorbed by its surroundings. A similar process takes places in the mind during *samadhi.* The mind will be 'coloured' by the object of meditation. As long as there is a flaw in the mind – an impurity or a distraction – there will be a distinction between the object and the mind, and complete absorption or identification will be impossible.

III, 4 Dharana, dhyana, *and* samadhi *together constitute* samyama.

When concentration on an object begins, and deepens into meditation, finally resulting in identification, the entire process is called *samyama*. For beginners this will take a long time, but adepts can perform *samyama* with lightning speed.

III, 5 *From the mastering of* samyama *follows higher knowledge.*

When *samyama* is practised, spiritual knowledge will dawn.

III, 7 Dharana, dhyana, *and* samadhi *are internal in relation to the five preceding steps.*

The first five steps of Yoga – abstention, observance, posture, breath control, and sense withdrawal – are called the outer stage, or *bahira anga*. The last three steps – concentration, meditation, and identification – are called the inner stage, or *antara anga*. Mental Yoga is therefore sometimes termed *antaranga,* or internal Yoga.

III, 8 *But even* dharana, dhyana, *and* samadhi *are external in relation to* nirbija samadhi.

Patanjali distinguishes between various forms of *samadhi*. If the concentration has begun on an object, be it concrete or abstract, the resulting *samadhi* falls under the heading *subija samadhi,* or *samadhi* with 'seed'. The 'seed', or *bija,* is the object. The knowledge gained in *sabija samadhi* in regard to the object of concentration, says Patanjali (I, 49), is of a higher kind than knowledge based on reasoning or testimony. The impression made on the mind during *sabija samadhi* is stronger than other impressions (I, 50).

In *nirbija,* or 'seedless', *samadhi* there is nothing in the highly trained and fully alert mind but consciousness and intense awareness of consciousness. Even the impressions resulting from *sabija samadhi* are suppressed (I, 51).

To arrive at *nirbija samadhi,* which is the higher of the two, one must be able to hold the mind in a prolonged thoughtless state, without any effort at all. In order to achieve this ability, the mind first has to go through a process called *nirodha parinama.* What this means will be explained in the next *sutra.*

III, 9 Nirodha parinama, *or suppression transformation, is the transformation through which the mind becomes accustomed to the moment of suppression that exists between the outgoing thought and the incoming thought.*

For the practice of *nirbija,* or objectless *samadhi,* it is necessary that the mind be held continuously in the state that prevails between two consecutive thoughts. There is a moment, after one thought has left the mind and before the next thought enters the field of consciousness, when there is no thought in the mind. At first this moment will be infinitely short, but by the suppression (*nirodha*) of the incoming thought, the moment between the thoughts is lengthened. At that particular time there is only consciousness in the mind. With practice, the mind gradually becomes capable of holding the conscious moment of no-thought with ease (III, 10). The required practice is, however, considerable.

The technique of concentrating on an object – intensified and resulting in *sabija samadhi,* or the *samadhi* with 'seed' – involves suppression of intruding thoughts. Therefore *sabija samadhi* is practised before *nirbija,* or seedless, *samadhi.*

IV, 29 *If one can remain disinterested even in the face of the greatest enlightenment, and one is able to practise the highest discrimination,* dharma-megha-samadhi *will follow.*

From the practice of the various yogic techniques so far described, the mind becomes a powerful instrument. Knowledge of ordinary things comes easily to one who has a perfectly trained mind, while higher knowledge is also attained (III, 5). The different types of *samadhi* result in deep insight. If a man is able to remain unaffected through these experiences, the highest *samadhi,* which is called *dharma-megha-samadhi,* will ensue. Whereas in previous *samadhis* he may have experienced a glimpse of the self, in *dharma-megha-samadhi* his mind becomes completely merged with the self. The experience makes him a yogi, and he is a changed man. He has attained self-realization. Nothing can affect him any more. He is freed from pain-bearing obstructions and the binding results of deeds (IV, 30). His state is called *kaivalya,* or independence.

CHAPTER THREE

Physical Yoga As Preparation

Through the science of physical Yoga, or Hatha Yoga, one can train the body to a high degree of efficiency, health, and beauty. These are attributes that almost everyone would like to possess. Hatha Yoga is an exacting, but interesting, discipline. However, the ultimate aim of physical Yoga is to prepare the mind for the difficult techniques of mental Yoga. The foremost classical textbook of Hatha Yoga is the *Hatha Yoga Pradipika,* by Svatmarama, an ancient work which opens with the declaration that Hatha Yoga is practised for the sake of Raja Yoga alone. Control of the body is but a preparation for mental control. Therefore students of physical Yoga will have a marked advantage when they begin their quest for victory over the mind.

The Raja Yoga student would be wise to practise some of the simple yet quite beneficial techniques of Hatha Yoga. He should lead a healthy, sensible life, and be moderate in his ways. The *Bhagavad Gita* states (VI, 16) that Yoga is verily not for him who eats or fasts too much, nor for him who sleeps too much or too little. The same sublime book condemns in later verses (XVII, 5-6) those who perform severe austerities and who torment the body. This should be a satisfactory refutation of the claims of those who say that one has to sleep on nails or starve oneself to emaciation in order to be a yogi.

The student should follow a wholesome diet, with the accent on natural foods, and he should avoid foods that are too salty or too spicy. He should also aim to strike a balance between sufficient exercise and sufficient rest.

Some of the basic Yoga postures, or *asanas,* and important breathing techniques are now described.

POSTURE OF COMPLETE RELAXATION
(SAVASANA)

Loosen all restrictive clothing. Lie on your back on a firm, flat surface. In *savasana,* the classical yogic relaxation posture, the arms are extended and away from the body, while the hands are open, palms up. The legs are apart, with the feet falling outwards. Keep the head straight, and close the eyes. The mouth is also closed, with the teeth slightly apart. When you are experienced in the art of relaxation – and an art it is – you will be able to 'let go' immediately, physically as well as mentally, without using any special technique. As a matter of fact, when you are really experienced, you will be relaxed all the time, whether you are lying in the posture under discussion, performing the headstand, weaving your way through dense traffic, or executing an intricate job. But for beginners there are several methods that will help greatly to bring about the desired physical and mental restfulness.

1. In the first method, we take an example from the animal kingdom. Picture a dog going to sleep. It will breathe in deeply, tense, and then let go suddenly with a contented sigh. Voila – instant relaxation!

Following this natural technique, breathe in deeply while lying in *savasana.* At the same time tense all the muscles in the body, every muscle you can think of. Hold everything for a few seconds, then let go suddenly with a contented sigh. Now feel that you are becoming so heavy that you are sinking into the floor. Every time you breathe out, you are sinking deeper.

If you want to, you can repeat the tensing and deep inhalation once or twice.

2. In the second method, we tense the different parts of the body separately. First tense all the muscles in the left leg while you breathe in deeply. Hold your breath and keep the leg tensed for a few seconds, then breathe out suddenly and release all the muscular contraction in the leg. Now direct your entire attention to that leg, and feel it become heavy and sink into

the floor. After ten or more seconds, repeat the process with the right leg. Then breathe in deeply, hold your breath and tense the abdominal muscles. Let go suddenly after a few seconds, and feel the abdomen sink lower every time you breathe out.

Next the left arm. Tense the whole arm as you breathe in deeply. Make a fist momentarily, hold your breath and muscular tension for a few seconds, then let go suddenly, and for ten or more seconds feel the arm sink into the floor. Do the same with the right arm.

Finally, breathe in deeply, then hold your breath and tense all the muscles in the neck. Let go suddenly, and feel the head become heavy and sink into the floor.

3. In the third method, you consciously withdraw all tension from the left leg, then from the right leg, and so on for every part of the body. Finally, relax the mind by visualizing a peace-inducing scene – for example, a beautiful garden, a sheltered, sunlit valley, or a deep blue sky.

Remain motionless in *savasana* for a period of five to ten minutes. After this refreshing rest, stand up slowly, breathe in deeply, and, with the arms above the head, stretch yourself elaborately.

The physiological benefits of *savasana* are, besides the obvious muscular and mental relaxation, a slowing down of the heart-beat and a lowering of the blood pressure.

THE EASY POSTURE (SUKHASANA)

An excellent posture for concentration and meditation is the easy posture, or *sukhasana*. The crossed legs are pulled close to the body, while the head, neck and spine are held erect. The open hands may be placed in the lap, one on top of the other, or the back of the wrists may be rested on the knees. Each person must find which is the more comfortable, and the least distracting, position for him. Some people find that when they sit on a hard surface in this posture, the top of the feet hurt. They may sit on a folded blanket. As soon as the legs begin to feel uncomfortable, the posture should be discontinued.

People who are of the opinion that the easy posture does

not live up to its name will often find the following posture more comfortable.

THE THUNDERBOLT POSTURE (VAJRASANA)

In the thunderbolt posture, or *vajrasana*, the feet are pointing backwards, and one sits on the heel. The hands are resting, palms down, on the thighs. As with the easy posture, the head, neck, and spine are held erect. There is one restriction, however. People with varicose veins in the legs should not sit in the thunderbolt posture for any length of time.

One must learn to sit still. When the body is still, the mind is inclined to follow suit.

Breathing is a function to which the student should give much thought and attention. We all know that the body must constantly receive a sufficient supply of oxygen. By deeply breathing in fresh air the Yoga student makes certain that the living cells of his body are well looked after. He can practise deep breathing in front of an open window as soon as he gets up in the morning, whenever he has the opportunity during the day, and especially at the start of his session of Yoga practice. Except for a few special exercises, he should always attempt to breathe in and out through the nose. In order to derive full benefit from breathing, the correct methods, as described below, should be learned.

ABDOMINAL BREATHING

Abdominal, or diaphragmatic, breathing is the way you used to breathe when you were a baby. Your memory may not go back that far; you probably have forgotten your original, and natural, breathing action, and therefore will have to learn it again. Women students will find it a little harder than their male counterparts to master again this beneficial breathing technique.

The diaphragm is a large dome-shaped muscle which separates the thorax from the abdomen. When at rest, it lies as a dome-shaped roof over the abdominal contents. When the muscle is contracted, it presses down on the abdominal organs, and these in turn force the abdomen out, making a 'big belly' as it were. The physiological benefit of diaphragmatic breathing, aside from supplying the system with plenty of fresh air, is that it gives a gentle massage to all the abdominal organs, thus aiding the blood circulation in that region.

At first the easiest way to practise abdominal breathing is to lie on your back, on the floor. No tight clothing should be worn. Place your fingers on your abdomen. Now breathe in deeply, at the same time trying to push your fingers up as high as possible with the abdomen. When you breathe out slowly, let the fingers fall down with the abdomen, then breathe in again, pushing the fingers up. Continue for a while, always breathing deeply and calmly. When it becomes easy to breathe in this manner, let your arms rest alongside the body, and try to push the abdomen up as you breathe in, without having the fingers on the abdomen. When you have sufficiently mastered this technique, try to do it while sitting up, and then while standing.

People with asthmatic tendencies will find abdominal breathing a most beneficial method of respiration.

THE COMPLETE BREATH

In the complete breath the entire breathing mechanism is brought into play. Every respiratory muscle is used, and every air cell of the lungs is filled with life-bringing air. The complete breath is a combination of three breathing methods: abdominal breathing, chest breathing, and upper breathing. Once you have mastered the abdominal breathing method, you are ready to commence the complete breath. It is best learned while lying down; later it can be practised while sitting, standing, or even while walking.

Lie on your back, with the arms stretched alongside the body. First take a deep abdominal breath. Now continue to breathe in while you fully expand the chest. At this stage the abdomen will fall back again, but that is how it should be. Just forget about the abdomen while you expand the chest. The third stage, upper breathing, is accomplished by slightly raising the shoulders and collarbones. Hold your breath for a few seconds, then breathe out slowly and evenly, paying no particular attention to shoulders, chest, or abdomen.

The inhalation is continuous, although at first the complete breath will consist of three distinct movements. Gradually the movements will flow into one another, giving the body a wave-like motion.

The benefits of deep breathing are not only physiological but also psychological. Deep breathing helps to banish fears, worries and anxieties. There is a close relationship between the breathing action and the state of the mind. When we are nervous, we breathe faster. By reversing the process – by purposely breathing more slowly – we will be able to calm the mind. There is an interesting Indian belief one would do well to remember. It holds that at birth man is allotted a specific number of breaths, and consequently by breathing more slowly, he will live longer. Great wisdom lies behind this seemingly simple idea.

CHAPTER FOUR

Pranayama
(Yogic Breathing)

Pranayama is the Sanskrit name for the yogic breathing techniques. The word means the restraining, or controlling, of the three parts of the breathing action : the inhalation, the retention, and the exhalation.

The breath is intimately connected with the mind. When we concentrate intensely on something – listening to a sudden sound, for example, or thinking very deeply – the breath is unconsciously suspended. We also find that when the mind is afflicted by fear or anger, the breath becomes irregular and rapid. Each of these instances demonstrates that the breath and the mind are interdependent. 'When the breath moves, the mind also moves' (*Hatha Yoga Pradipika*, II, 2).

In order to control the restless activity of the mind, the Yoga student should learn to regulate the breath.

Once the student is able to sit comfortably in a firm posture, and has learned to moderate his eating habits, he can commence the practice of *pranayama*.

The surface on which he sits should not be too hard for comfort. Yogic breathing exercises should not be practised for some time after a meal.

The nasal passages should first be cleaned. This can be accomplished by means of a handkerchief or, more traditionally, by drawing up water through each nostril from the hollow of the hand or from a bowl. The water is drawn up through one nostril until it comes out at the back of the throat and is expelled through the mouth. As this practice is helpful in preventing colds and in clearing the head, the student would do well to perform it every day. At first the water touching the nerves at the top of the back of the nasal passage may cause a strange sensation, but one soon becomes accustomed to it. One may practise while taking a shower; when the head is tilted slightly backwards, the water will run into the nose. People who suffer from sinus trouble should not practise this technique.

The regular practice of *pranayama* helps the student to over-come all fears, even the fear of death, according to the *Hatha Yoga Pradipika* (II, 39), the leading treatise on Hatha Yoga, Nevertheless, the practice of *pranayama* should never be forced. The *Hatha Yoga Pradipika* warns: 'Just as the lion, the ele-phant and the tiger are tamed only very gradually, so the breath is controlled by slow degrees, otherwise it kills (harms) the practitioner' (II, 15).

The warning is clear enough – you should never strain your-self during the practice of *pranayama*. Svatmarama, the author of the above work, states further: 'Carefully one should exhale air; carefully inhale it; carefully hold it' (II, 17).

During yogic breathing the lungs are not held completely empty – after all, air means life. In this regard it is pointedly stated: 'As long as the air stays in the body, so long there is life' (II, 3).

In *pranayama* the ratio between inhalation and exhalation is 1:2. In other words the exhalation is always twice as long as the inhalation; if the inhalation lasts two seconds, the exhalation lasts four seconds. The breath is never held any longer than is comfortable. If retention causes even the slightest discomfort, the purpose of the practice of *pranayama* is de-feated. To establish the correct ratio between inhalation, reten-tion, and exhalation, the student would be wise to practise rhythmic breathing for a few weeks before trying to master the *pranayamas*.

RHYTHMIC BREATHING

Beginners can first practise the ratio between inhalation, retention, and exhalation as 1:2:2. Breathe in deeply for two seconds, hold your breath for four seconds, then breathe out slowly for four seconds. Once this becomes easy, you may breathe in for three seconds, hold your breath for six seconds, then breathe out in six seconds. Instead of mentally counting off the seconds, you could ·count the heartbeats by holding the pulse.

More advanced students should aim for a ratio between inhalation, retention, and exhalation of $1:4:2$. If the inhalation lasts two seconds, the retention should last for eight seconds, and the exhalation for four seconds. Later, the inhalation can be for three seconds, retention for twelve seconds, and the exhalation for six seconds. Gradually the duration of each part of the respiration can be lengthened, as long as the ratio $1:4:2$ is maintained, until at last the retention is for sixty-four seconds (the duration of inhalation and exhalation then being sixteen seconds and thirty-two seconds, respectively).

The Sanskrit word for inhalation is *puraka;* for breath retention, *kumbhaka;* for exhalation, *rechaka.* Instead of counting seconds, or pulse beats, the able student may also mentally recite the syllables of the above Sanskrit words. While breathing in, slowly recite *pu-ra-ka;* while holding air confined, mentally recite four times *kum-bha-ka;* while breathing out, twice recite *re-cha-ka.* With practice the number of repetitions can gradually be increased.

ALTERNATE BREATHING

The student is traditionally advised to practise alternate breathing before performing any of the other *pranayamas.* Alternate breathing is also highly recommended as a method for calming the nerves.

In alternate breathing we inhale and exhale alternately through the left and right nostril. First try the following technique for closing off either nostril : the index and middle fingers of the right hand are placed along the length of the nose, so that the right nostril can be closed comfortably by pressing the thumb against the side of the nose, and the left nostril by pressing with the little and ring fingers.

Alternate breathing commences by breathing in through the left nostril only. Both nostrils are then firmly closed, and the breath is held according to the practitioner's ability. The mind is fixed on the space between the eyebrows. When it is no longer comfortable to hold the breath, the air is expelled slowly through the right nostril only. As soon as the exhalation has been completed, one breathes in deeply again through the same nostril, i.e., the right nostril. Breath retention is followed by exhalation and inhalation through the left nostril, and so on. Always breathe out and in through the one nostril, keeping the air confined as long as is comfortable, then breathing out and in through the other nostril, and continuing for as long as desired.

Alternate breathing and rhythmic breathing can be combined so that they make one exercise.

SUN BREATH (SURYA BHEDANA)

This *pranayama* exercise involves inhalation through the right nostril only. The air coming in through that nostril is regarded as a symbol for the sun (*surya*).

Breathe in slowly but deeply through the right nostril, then retain the breath for as long a period as possible without discomfort. During the breath retention the mind is focused on the space between the eyebrows. The exhalation is through the left nostril only, and is slow and even.

VICTORIOUS BREATH (UJJAYI)

Breathe in deeply and forcefully through both nostrils. The rate at which the air is made to stream into the lungs should be uniform. Hold the breath as long as is comfortable, and focus the mind on the space between the eyebrows. Exhalation is through the mouth. Holding the mouth as if whistling, breathe out slowly and evenly, making a soft sound at a steady pitch. Continue with the even exhalation until the lungs are completely empty. If the breath has been held too long, you will have difficulty executing the exhalation as prescribed, or you may have to gasp for air at the end of the whistling exhalation. Should this happen, rest for a moment, then start again, this time making sure that the breath is not held too long.

One may also practise *ujjayi* by exhaling through the left nostril only, instead of through the mouth.

HISSING SOUND BREATH (SITKARI)

Sitkari is performed by sucking air in through the mouth while the teeth are clenched and the tongue is held suspended so that it does not touch the inside of the mouth. While inhaling, a hissing sound is made, and attention is concentrated on the cool feeling on the tongue. Then the mouth is closed, the breath held for as long as is comfortable, and the mind focused on the space between the eyebrows. The air is expelled slowly through the nose.

The *Hatha Yoga Pradipika* (II, 54–6) promises as a tempting added benefit that *sitkari* makes the practitioner next to the god of love in beauty and the subject of adoration by the yoginis (female yogis are sometimes called yoginis). Although not mentioned, it can be presumed that, conversely, it makes the female practitioner adorable in the eyes of the yogis. However, as the aim of *pranayama* is to calm the mind, it may be wiser not to think of *sitkari* as a path to beauty and adoration by the opposite sex.

COOLING BREATH (SITALI)

This breathing exercise is similar to *sitkari,* the only difference being in the way mouth and tongue are held during the inhalation. In *sitali* the tongue protrudes from the lips. The mouth is half open in such a way that the hissing sound is still made. The breath is retained as long as is comfortable. Exhalation is through the nose.

BELLOW BREATH (BHASTRIKA)

A rapid succession of about ten quick exhalations, each followed by an equally quick inhalation, is performed through the nose. This part of the *bhastrika pranayama* makes a sound similar to that produced by the bellows of a blacksmith. The last inhalation of the series is very forceful and deep. Then the breath is suspended as long as can be done with comfort, while the mind is focused on the space between the eyebrows. Breathe out slowly and evenly through both nostrils.

As a variation, the inhalation series may be done through one nostril only (either the left or the right nostril), while the exhalation is done through the right nostril instead of through both nostrils.

Bhastrika is a very intense exercise. Therefore beginners should perform this *pranayama* for no more than three rounds, and then take a short rest. With progress, the number of quick inhalations and exhalations can be increased from about ten up to twenty or thirty, and the complete *pranayama* can be practised more often.

INTERNAL SOUNDS BREATH (BHRAMARI)

The ears are sealed off by the hands. The inhalation and exhalation are both through the nose. Breathe in forcefully. During the breath retention, listen to the various internal sounds of the body. The inhalation and exhalation produce a sound similar to that of the humming of bees; the forceful inhalation sounds like the male bee, and the slow exhalation like the female bee.

Bhramari is best practised at night, in quiet surroundings.

SWOONING BREATH (MURCHHA)

Breathe in deeply through the nose. Press the chin firmly into the jugular notch and hold the breath as long as is comfortable. The mind is concentrated on the space between the eyebrows. Exhale slowly while the chin is still firmly pressed to the chest. During the inhalation the head is kept up. The chin lock, which is applied during the retention and the exhalation, is called *jalandhara bandha*. Its physiological benefits are the exercise of the neck muscles, improvement of blood circulation around the throat, and strengthening of the thyroid and parathyroid glands.

Beginners may find it easier at first to apply the chin lock during the retention of the breath only.

CHAPTER FIVE

Concentration and Mental Exercises

Concentration is the focusing of all mental energies upon one object or one idea. In everyday life we all concentrate at times. With protruding tongue, we try to put a thread through the eye of a needle. Drawing a picture, we are oblivious of everything else. With extreme alertness we manoeuvre our car through an area congested with traffic. This type of concentration can be classified as external, since it is something in the external world that draws and holds our attention.

Dharana, or yogic concentration, is internal. The process takes place entirely within the field of consciousness, and is directed by the will. In external concentration the job being performed, or the picture being looked at, demands our attention. There is no conscious effort at concentration; it simply happens. Internal concentration is much more difficult. Here the mind is commanded by the will to hold its attention to something which is purposely placed in the field of consciousness. The Yoga student must learn to hold his unwavering attention to anything he decides to concentrate upon, whether it is something important or something insignificant. He must be able to bring his mind into focus whenever he decides to do so, and then he must be able to sustain this singleness of concentration for any length of time.

For the untrained mind conscious concentration is extremely difficult. After long periods of chaotic freedom, the mind does not take kindly to discipline. Often it will react violently, behaving as if it were a disturbed hornets' nest. Try not to think, and at once a host of thoughts will invade the mind. Attempt to concentrate on one idea, and in quick succession unconnected thoughts will be clamouring for attention. If we try to slow down the thinking process, thoughts will begin to race through the mind at a frantic pace. Gradually, however, the mind can be transformed into a useful and effective instrument. One must practise regularly and diligently.

To start with, one should try to concentrate on concrete objects. Too many difficulties are encountered by the novice if he begins with abstract and complicated ideas. One should select something simple, and then try to hold it in the mind for as long as possible. Alien thoughts will come into the field of consciousness, but one must dispassionately attach the attention once more to the object of concentration. Above all, one must remain calm. If one becomes angry because concentration seems impossible, matters will only be made worse. A detached perseverance is essential. One takes the mind by the hand, as one would a young child, and gently guides it again and again to the chosen object.

There may be times when a thought continues to intrude, perhaps with such annoying persistency that it seems impossible to concentrate. If that is the case, one could make that particular thought the subject of the concentration practice. The point is not to become annoyed. Another way of dealing with the intruding thought is to promise oneself to dwell upon this thought at some future time.

Mind-wandering can be arrested. There is plenty of time for daydreaming, but not during concentration practice. Often you will begin to think of, perhaps, a tree, and a few minutes later you will suddenly discover that you are thinking about something totally different. If this is so, firmly tell yourself that that will be the end of the reverie, and gently bring the attention of the mind once more to the object of concentration.

Although the mind should not be allowed to drift away, it may be permitted to think of direct associations with the object under consideration, as long as it constantly returns to that object. The mind moves from the central idea to explore different aspects of it. In this way everything that is relevant to the main theme is placed under a mental microscope.

If you try too hard to concentrate, the opposite of the desired result is apt to ensue. Examples of this abound in everyday life. Try too hard to speak correctly, and you will begin to make mistakes. Try too hard to draw a perfect picture, and you may fail dismally. If there is too much tension behind the effort to concentrate, the endeavour will be wasted. Just as the physical eye does not get tired if it operates without strain, so the mind must remain calm for efficient concentration.

The student should not be discouraged if at first his efforts at concentration seem to bear little fruit. Consistent practice will enhance the mind's ability to focus its powers of attention. With practice, concentration can be made a fine art. The student will be able to single out a thought or idea, and hold it in his mind without any deviation or interruption for as long as he likes. He will attain great knowledge about whatever he focuses his attention upon. He will be able to bring any thought into his mind, hold it there for examination, then dismiss the thought and at once be ready to give the same intense attention to the next idea. When he can do this, he will also be able to banish thoughts altogether, and hold his mind in the unmodified state called *nirodha,* which means restraint, or control.

In order to improve the faculty of concentration various mental exercises can be practised. If possible, the student should set aside some time each day for this purpose. It is recommended that the exercises be practised at a set time, preferably early 'in the morning, but if this presents difficulties, the time that suits the student best is the best time. Once he is somewhat more experienced, the student may be able to use odd moments – of commuting or waiting – which might otherwise be wasted, for the practice of some of the simpler mental techniques.

MENTAL EXERCISES

At first, it is advisable to practise the mental exercises under the most favourable circumstances. One should be alone, and one should know that one will not be disturbed for some time. There should be no draught in the room; the light should not be too bright; the temperature should be agreeable. The room should preferably be sparsely furnished, and, if possible, one should sit facing a bare wall. Most exercises are more easily performed with the eyes closed. One should not practise just after a large meal, because the immediate effects of too much food are a slight discomfort and sleepiness.

It is very difficult for the novice to step out of the often hectic and rushed life of the world and, without a transition period, enter the world of the mind. Therefore, if you are a student of physical Yoga, practise this before you commence the mental techniques. If not, it is still advisable to practise some physical relaxation first, to do a few deep breathing and stretching exercises (after having attended to the demands of the excretory system). It is not good, at least for beginners, to perform mental exercise while physically or mentally tired. Concentration is too demanding. Also, the mind should not be occupied with any worldly or emotional problems.

The mental exercises are preceded by *pranayama,* or yogic breathing. Regulation of the breath quiets the mind. When one feels that the mind is sufficiently calmed, one is ready. After the practice of *pranayama,* no attention at all is paid to the breath.

The posture assumed should be firm and comfortable. If the mind is distracted by bodily aches and pains, or even slight discomforts, concentration will be extremely difficult. If one can sit comfortably in the easy posture, or *sukhasana*, one will find that posture very useful. Others will find the thunderbolt posture, or *vajrasana,* more pleasant. One may also sit on a stool, keeping the head up, the back straight, and the legs together. The feet are planted firmly on the floor, the hands are resting on the thighs. One may also try to practise some mental exercises while lying on the back in *savasana.*

In the beginning the concentration exercises cannot be practised for a very long period. The early sessions should last about ten minutes, no more. Some people can concentrate for longer periods than others, however, so there is no set rule.

One should practise with great diligence. Intensity of effort is far more important than duration of practice. The order in which the techniques are given is suggested, but one may begin with any exercise that appeals. The whole time may be spent on the practice of one exercise, or one can do several during one session. Once a particular mental exercise has been mastered to a degree, one may commence the next. It is best to keep on practising the selected exercise till some measure of success has been achieved. Gradually the duration of each exercise is lengthened.

TRATAKA

A beneficial and often practised exercise is *trataka,* or staring. It is one of the six *kriyas,* or cleansing duties, and it helps to bring about stillness of the mind.

One gazes without blinking at a point or a small object for one or two minutes, as long as one can without straining the eyes and eye muscles. It is better to close the eyes and rest them when there is discomfort, and then repeat the exercise, than to hold the object in view for too long. These directions apply to all eye exercises. With practice, the duration of each uninterrupted gazing period can be lengthened considerably.

One may also look steadily at the point of the nose. This ancient method helps to strengthen the eyes. Occasional squinting is not harmful to the eyes as is sometimes thought, but, on the contrary, it will improve them.

Similar to the nasal gaze is the frontal gaze, in which one directs the eyes to the point midway between the eyebrows. As this is rather strenuous on the eye muscles, the eyes should be rested as soon as the need is felt.

Another technique which helps to steady the mind and strengthen the eyes is that of gazing at a lighted candle. This is performed in a dark room where there is no draught, otherwise the flame will move and this will spoil the effect of the exercise. One sits about three or four feet away from the candle, and gazes fixedly at the flame. When it is time to stop, the cupped hands are placed over the closed eyes. The after-image of the flame will still be visible, and one may continue to look at this as a further aid to stopping the mind from wandering.

VISUALIZATION

Visualization is the calling up of an image with such concentration and imagination that the picture seen with the mind's eye is as vivid as the actual object would be. If one were to evoke the image of a rose, one would see the magnificent flower clearly projected on the screen of the mind. One would be able to admire its gracious form and its beautiful colour, and one would see the picture in such detail that the number of petals could be counted, and the thorns on the stem distinguished. The whole visualization would be so life-like that one might even imagine smelling the flower's exquisite fragrance.

TRAVELLING TO A DISTANT PLACE

With intense concentration, the power of visualization can be applied so strongly that one can mentally transport oneself to any place on earth and experience the sensation of being in the locality of one's choice as if one were really there. If the student should decide to go to a beautiful spot in a natural setting – perhaps near a waterfall – he would close his eyes and, leaving the present surroundings, travel with the speed of light to the distant goal. Once having arrived there, he would visualize his presence at the peaceful site to such a degree that he could hear the soothing chatter of the water, and the calls of exotic birds; he would breathe in the healthy air, and feel kissed by the warm rays of the sun.

When the student reluctantly opens his eyes at the end of the exercise, it will come as quite a surprise to him to find himself still in the same place from whence he had set out.

COUNTING ONE'S BLESSINGS

There is much in life to be thankful for. Now the student stops and fully realizes this. He may commence the exercise by reflecting upon the senses, and thinking how wondrous they are, and what a great blessing it is to possess those five faculties. To be healthy is a wonderful gift, something to be very grateful for. It is far more important than being wealthy, or than attaining high social standing. Health is a precious treasure, and the Yoga student is thankful for the science of Hatha Yoga which helps him to become healthy and to stay healthy. It is wonderful to have control over one's body, and, to the student of Raja Yoga, even more wonderful to have control over the mind. The Jnana Yoga student marvels at the exalted wisdom taught by the Indian sages of old.

Each one of us has had many things happen to him for which he should be extremely grateful. In the exercise of counting his blessings the student dwells upon these things, and he carries the feeling of gratitude with him into his daily life.

LISTENING TO THE TICKING OF A CLOCK

In a very quiet room in which there is a softly ticking clock, attempt to hear the sound made by the clock from some distance away. Direct your full attention to listening. Once you can discern it, you may make the exercise more difficult by sitting farther away.

Instead of a clock, you may also use a wrist watch for the purpose of training. First place your watch close to your ear. When you can hear the workings of its delicate mechanism, rest your wrist on your shoulder, and see if you can still hear the soft ticking. Once your ears discover the near-silent sound, move your hand lower and place it on the arm just under the shoulder, and then further down.

OBSERVATION

For the observation exercise one may concentrate on any given object. First let it be a simple thing, such as an apple. The object – in this case the apple – is placed at eye level, at such a distance that continuous observation of it does not strain the eyes. Once settled down, one begins to look at the apple with special interest. Notice all its peculiarities in detail. Study its shape and size. Observe the different shades of colour in its skin. Study the texture of the skin. See whether it is smooth or slightly dented and discoloured. Look carefully at the protruding stalk, and at how the apple is shaped around it. Besides the visual observation, try to detect the object's fragrance.

Attention should be concentrated on the apple until its every feature is firmly imprinted on the mind, so that one can see it just as clearly with the eyes closed as with the eyes open.

OBSERVATION AND RECALL

After closely observing an object, one closes one's eyes and attempts to reconstruct it in the mind, giving meticulous attention to even the most minute detail. As before, one may use any given object, or one can observe one's surroundings and, after careful examination, mentally reproduce them. If sitting outside, one recalls the scenery, and if indoors, one recalls the room and its contents.

With the practice of this exercise, the powers of observation and memory are increased. In everyday life one will discover many interesting facts about common objects. One will learn to go through life with eyes wide open and become increasingly aware of the great wonders to be seen everywhere.

THINKING ABOUT AN OBJECT AND ITS ASSOCIATIONS

In this exercise one selects an object for practice, and then thinks of all the things that can be associated with it. If an apple is the chosen object, one is here not so much concerned with its appearance as with thoughts about it, such as where the apple came from; how it came into one's possession; the people who grow apples; those who deal in apples; he who is kept away if one apple a day is eaten; the different kinds of apples; the various flavours to be found in the fruit; its many uses in cooking; in its role in Swiss legend; how its simple act of falling from a tree is said to have inspired a great scientist; how useful it is in mental exercises, and on and on.

THOUGHT OBSERVATION

Here, thoughts are allowed to come and go as they please, while the student steps out of his mind, as it were, and becomes an objective spectator. He dissociates himself from his thoughts, gives his mind free rein, and attentively observes the ensuing mental activity. He watches the incessant parade of thoughts passing through his mind in quick succession. If hideous thoughts happen to come into the field of consciousness, he should not be appalled, but should remain a dispassionate observer. He may be surprised at the thoughts that come into his mind; he may have been of the opinion that it was impossible for him to have such thoughts. Sitting calmly, he should realize that repulsive ideas are but manifestations of the lower nature, which he is striving to overcome.

At first the mind, freed from all controls, will race on, but gradually its activity will diminish, its caprices become less violent.

At the end of the exercise, the practitioner may reflect back on his various thoughts, recognizing each for what it was. He may also try to discover a pattern in their coming and going, and attempt to see how the different thoughts were associated.

SLOWING DOWN MENTAL ACTIVITY

Physical relaxation and mental relaxation are two states that accompany each other. By first resting the body, and then practising *pranayama* (yogic breathing) for a period, the student prepares himself best for the state of mental quiescence. Thoughts are crossing the mind, but they do so in slow motion, without the rapid succession and sudden change of subject that normally takes place in the untrained mind. When mental activity is slowed down, the mind can be compared to a vast blue sky, and the occasional thoughts to isolated small clouds passing overhead. The student can actually think of a blue sky, and with his mind's eye see a small white cloud lazily drifting across the firmament. He then attaches a thought to that cloud, lets it slowly pass through his mind, and in time allows it to disappear beyond the horizon. As he watches the sky, another thought-cloud appears, and the restful exercise proceeds.

SUPPRESSION OF THOUGHTS

Thoughts continuously enter the mind. This process can be halted, and the present exercise is an attempt in this direction. The practitioner exercises extreme mental alertness; as soon as a thought crops up, he resolutely pushes it back. The student will find that thoughts come at the mind from all angles, as it were, and he must remain ever watchful; he should regard the oncoming thoughts as intruders which he has to bar from the field of consciousness. Repressing thoughts is a very demanding exercise, and before long the mind will become tired. As soon as this happens, thoughts should once more be freely allowed to enter the mind. After sufficient rest, the exercise is recommenced

Concentrating on thoughts about only one object or subject may be difficult, but endeavouring not to think at all is even harder. Although an adept in Yoga can wipe his mind clear of thought at will, and without effort, beginners will more likely encounter great difficulty in halting the compelling stream of thoughts racing through their restless minds. Therefore they may at this early stage call in physical aids in order to suppress thoughts and to maintain for a period a state of blankness of mind. They will find this condition easier to achieve if they breathe in deeply, hold the breath, close the eyes, and then look up – the eyes remaining closed – at a point midway between the eyebrows. An additional aid to students is the application of the tongue lock, called the *khecari mudra,* in which the tongue is folded and made to reach back as far as possible towards the throat. The *mudra* should be held only for the duration of the breath retention.

CONCENTRATION ON THE BREATH

Breathing calmly, focus the entire attention of the mind on the light flow of air that comes in and goes out through the nostrils. Breathing in, you will feel the cool incoming air fill the nasal cavity. When you breathe deeper, but still slowly, you will be able to follow the stream of air as it reaches the throat, and even further, right into the larynx.

At first, concentration on the breath may strike you as an insignificant technique, but a' little practice will soon convince you of the profound stabilizing effect it has on the mind. It is an exercise that can be practised with beneficial results in time of tension, and is also of great use to people who suffer from insomnia.

CALM BREATH

Join the word 'calm' to the incoming breath, making the

word last until the end of the inhalation. Then again think 'calm' to the outgoing breath, making it last for the duration of the exhalation. You are constantly and rhythmically repeating 'calm, calm, calm, calm . . .'.

COUNTING BREATHS

A simple yet very soothing exercise which requires, and further develops, concentration of mind is the counting of breaths. While sitting quietly and breathing calmly, mentally count every inhalation. Continue to breathe evenly and rhythmically, oblivious to the outside world, and undisturbed by thoughts that may try to intrude into your mind. Count up to one hundred, then move a bead on your *mala* (rosary), or use your fingers for counting every hundred. Alternatively, you may make a mark on a piece of paper with a pen or pencil.

If you become distracted and the count is broken, make a mental note of the number at which you lost count. With practice you will be able to reach a higher total without being disturbed. Of course it would be absolutely contrary to the whole purpose of the exercise if you were to breathe faster in order to increase the total number of breaths counted.

DIRECTING THE FLOW OF THE BREATH

In the alternate yogic breathing exercise the stream of air is directed first through one nostril, and then through the other, by alternately pressing thumb or little and ring fingers against the side of the nose. Alternate nostril breathing can also be attempted without physically closing off one nostril. Another difference in the purely mental technique is that the breath is not held.

The mental method of directing the nasal flow of air requires complete concentration. When breathing in through the left nostril first, the entire consciousness is focused on the air coming in through that side of the nose. The mind is not allowed to feel anything else. The same applies when the air is expelled through the right nostril, and then brought in again.

C

PRANIC BREATH

People with a Western education know that when they breathe in fresh air their systems take in oxygen. The absorption of the oxygen into the blood stream occurs in the fine capillaries of the lungs. The blood distributes the life-giving element throughout the body. In this way all living cells of the organism are supplied with the oxygen they need in order to continue functioning.

Thousands of years ago, yogis evolved the theory that the atmosphere contained a vital force, which they called *Prana,* and which they saw as a universal and fundamental energy. *Prana,* they taught, is everywhere, and in everything; it is the basic force that animates all matter. The force that causes the planets to move is *Prana,* and *Prana* is likewise the energy that accounts for all action of and within the human body, not only on the physical plane, but also in the field of mental activity. Muscular movement is a grosser manifestation of *Prana,* while thought and will are more subtle expressions.

The Yoga student may regard *Prana* as concentrated energy, present everywhere. The oxygen he breathes in is a form of *Prana,* as is that vital force that energizes his nervous system. In this manner the esoteric Eastern explanation is aligned with the scientific Western point of view. In the *Pranic* breath the practitioner feels that he deeply inhales an abundance of *Prana.* The breath is held for as long as is comfortable, and during retention the vital force is visualized as moving throughout the body, vitalizing every part. Should a particular organ need special attention it is singled out and mentally given an extra helping of the cosmic energy. Students intent on increasing their powers of thought can send an ample flow of *Prana* to the brain.

FEELING INCREASED WARMTH OR COLD

Although the surrounding temperature remains the same, the practitioner becomes either warmer or colder. In a gradual mental process he can imagine that he is sitting in the sun, whose solar rays are warming his body, or that he is sitting in front of a fire whose heat is enveloping him. He can also feel that the *Prana* he is inhaling is generating a glow inside his physical abode.

The imagined increase in warmth can be felt to such an extent that one actually begins to perspire. Likewise, a drop in bodily temperature can be felt if one thinks oneself either partly or totally submerged in cold water, or surrounded by ice, or shut in a freezing chamber.

SOLAR PLEXUS CHARGING

In the upper part of the abdomen, on either side of the spinal column, lies the solar plexus, a compact bundle of nerves connected with the sympathetic nervous system. It is a large and important nerve centre, situated as it is in a dominant position in the middle of the body, from whence it governs the vital organs. The solar plexus has been identified with the yogic *manipura chakra,* a subtle centre within the spinal column at the level of the navel, and it is seen as a storehouse for *Pranic* energy.

While breathing in slowly and evenly, visualize a golden stream of *Prana* which is all around you in the atmosphere. Feel it enter the head at the crown, and consciously direct this stream of life-bringing energy to the solar plexus. While breathing out, circulate the *Prana* in and around the solar plexus, increasing the speed of the circulation with every new exhalation.

THE POSITIVE BREATH

We decide on a positive quality we would like to possess. It may be health, or it may be a mental quality. If it is health we have decided upon, we breathe in deeply through the nose, and feel that we inhale abundant health. If we have decided upon a moral or mental quality, we likewise feel it stream into us as we inhale deeply. The quality chosen can be calmness, or willpower, or detachment, or selflessness, or any other characteristic we know to be positive from the yogic point of view.

EXPELLING UNDESIRABLE CHARACTERISTICS

Most people would readily admit that they have some weakness in their mental make-up which they would rather be
without. Life can appear complicated, and the forces and
temptations arrayed against one can seem overwhelming. If
there is a particular flaw in your character which has repeatedly
been your downfall in the past, and which very likely will be a
hindrance to progress in your programme for self-development
and Yoga, select this fault which you want to shed, isolate it
from yourself, and use it in practising this method of throwing
off undesirable characteristics.

There are two ways of doing this exercise. The first involves
breathing in and out through the nose, and feeling that with
each forceful exhalation you are expelling the unwanted quality
through the nostrils. If your feelings about the detested fault are
very strong – it has been annoying you for too long – use the
second method, and expel it forcefully and contemptuously
through the anus with every exhalation.

REFLECTION AT THE END OF THE DAY

This is a mental exercise to be practised before retiring. The
student is to think back on the day just passed, asking himself
honestly whether he acted throughout as a good Yoga student
should. Life contains many pitfalls for the unwary traveller
but this is no excuse for the person intent on mental progress.
If he went wrong in some situation during the day just past
the student should, without evasion, think back on it and ask
himself why he erred. He should examine the reasons for this
temporary failure, and finally he should mentally relive the
whole scene, only this time conducting himself as master of
himself, as he should have done then.

At the conclusion of the exercise, the student should resolve
to overcome any weakness or faults he may have shown.

The above techniques can also be adapted to shortcomings
of the more distant past.

After considering your yogic training up till now and assessing
which stage you have reached, decide what you have yet to

achieve. In order to get an idea of what remains to be done, read this book right through, and then map out your future training programme accordingly. Take into account any restricting circumstances you are likely to encounter, as well as personal relationships you will have to reckon with. Determine which things might, for no good reason, take up too much of your precious time and mental energy, and resolve to drop them. In the firm assurance that the goal – Yoga – is worth any sacrifice, decide how much time you are going to devote each day to your self-training. Remember that the more you practice, the more you will benefit and progress. Reflect on any plans you might have for your worldly life, and see that they fit in with your Yoga programme. Sincerely resolve to eliminate anything that might be detrimental to a serious Yoga student. Plan your strategy as a general would prepare for battle.

RECALL

The number of facts stored away in the memory is staggering. With a calm mind one can recall scenes from early childhood, relations with father and mother, first school days, teachers, friends, and occurrences throughout one's life, many of which were thought long forgotten. However, if one tries too hard to remember something in particular, the task becomes increasingly difficult, until at last the mind becomes overburdened and temporarily 'blacks out', or 'freezes'; all its activities are halted for a moment, and one can neither remember, nor even think. The opposite is true when the mind is placid – the calmer the mind, the more one can recapture. Therefore an absolutely tranquil state is essential for maximum results. Only when the mind is as calm as a cloudless blue sky is it fully receptive to messages coming in from the subconscious.

There is so much filed away in the memory system that any item at all can be used as a subject for an exercise in recall. The method is first to decide what one is going to recollect, and then purposefully activate the particular *samskaras* (memory traces). If the item one is trying to remember is elusive, remaining just beyond the border of the mind, one should momentarily discontinue the mental search. This can be done directly by simply disregarding the whole matter, but many untrained people will find this very hard. An indirect technique, namely the focusing of the attention of the mind on something totally different, is most helpful here. The subject one uses to lure the mind away can be a set subject especially selected for this purpose – one which can be used again and again, such as a simple figure or drawing, or a peaceful landscape into which one makes one's mental retreat. Success through this method however, is only obtained through a one hundred per cent effort. If part of the mind is still busily engaged in the search for the elusive fact, all efforts at deliberate distraction will be futile. One should at the time not even be aware of the reason for concentrating upon something else. If one is continually aware that the mind is being led in another direction, and continuously checking to see if the technique is working, one will not be successful in either exercise.

In the Recall exercise, it is a good idea to choose a simple and insignificant subject for recollection. For example, one could try to remember the contents of the morning's newspaper. If one has not seen that paper, one can try to recollect what was in the last paper or magazine one read. One may also retrace one's actions during that day from the moment of rising or the activities of the previous day or of any other day.

The student who has fully read this section of the book can try to remember as many mental exercises as possible, and if he has studied the Yoga philosophy, he can try to recite from memory some of the profound utterances of the Indian sages.

RELIVING PAST EXPERIENCES

The reliving of past experiences is an exercise closely allied to the Recall exercise. It can be regarded as a natural extension of that technique. After deciding which experience one is going to revive, the particular *samskaras* (memory traces) are activated and the entire consciousness is focused on the messages coming into the mind. When there are neither external nor internal distractions, the whole experience to be remembered is mentally re-enacted in depth. The student goes back in time, traverses great distances, and plays out complete scenes from his earlier life. He talks to old friends, and experiences once more anguish or pleasure, as the case may be.

Instead of reliving past experiences, the process may be reversed and *future experiences* lived – if the same resolution is employed. Sitting calmly on his mat, the trained Yoga student can, should he choose to do so, go anywhere, meet anybody, and do anything. He realizes more than anyone else that it is 'all in the mind'. He can even, as a mental exercise, leave his own body and assume the physical and psychological identity of another person, experiencing that person's reactions to life.

DISCOVERING THE GOOD SIDE OF AN OCCURRENCE

The occurrence chosen for practice in this particular exercise is an event previously thought unpleasant. The aim is to reflect deeply in order to discover any good aspect that a given unfavourable experience may possibly have had.

Ask yourself whether the experience taught you something and made you a wiser person, more mature, more realistic. That is what life is – a succession of pleasant and unpleasant experiences. Sometimes the former have the upper hand, sometimes the latter. Whatever took place had to happen, in obedience to the Law of *Karma* (the Law of Cause and Effect). Everything that happens – be it in the past, the present, or the future – has a cause, and cause and effect follow one another in relentless sequence. To call an occurrence 'bad' only reflects one's mental attitude at the time. Through Yoga one learns to look at things in a more detached way. Everything in the sense-perceived world is subject to change, and the sooner one realizes and accepts this, the quicker one will progress.

THINKING OF SOMEONE YOU DISLIKE

Thoughts are centred on a person for whom you have no particular liking, or one whom you detest. Instead of dwelling on what you have always regarded as this individual's bad points, you are now to concentrate on any positive qualities he may have. If you cannot discover any, you had better try harder. Imagine that this person you so dislike is a blood relation whom you are called upon to defend against an injustice.

When being critical, you should always bear in mind that had you been that person, and had you encountered exactly the same circumstances, you might have behaved in exactly the same way. If you are in a critical mood, analyse your thoughts and motives, and ask yourself whether the fault may lie with you. Then replace criticism of others with understanding.

Conclude the present exercise by mentally sending a message of good will and love to the person who provided you with a subject for concentration.

If you cannot possibly think of anyone you dislike, you will have to forsake this exercise. However, you may congratulate yourself, for you are well advanced on the path to peace. To the yogi there is no such thing as an enemy. All men and women are his beloved brothers and sisters. He has in his heart an abundant love for the whole of Creation.

THINKING OF A SUBJECT YOU DISLIKE

If there is a subject you do not like to think about, for the purpose of this exercise *do* think about it. Your mind must be strong enough to think about anything. There is no need to mention to anyone those thoughts you resent, but dwell upon them in the solitude of your own mind. Perhaps there are thoughts that you had pushed back into the far corners of your subconscious, and these thoughts have the habit of coming into view at the most unexpected moments. Bring them up deliberately and analyse your feelings about them.

INCREASING SIZE OF BODY

Sitting quietly with your eyes closed, feel your body grow larger every time you inhale, as if it were a balloon being blown up. Feel yourself increase in height, and simultaneously feel your chest expand. The exercise should be a one hundred per cent mental effort, because as soon as your concentration is disturbed only slightly you will have to start all over again.

Keep on blowing yourself up until your head touches the ceiling of the room; after that, your chest expands further until your body completely fills the room, to the farthest corner. Once you have achieved this, you have performed the first stage of the exercise. You may discontinue the exercise here, and mentally deflate your body in one exhalation.

For the second stage, continue to bring air into your body with deep gulps. The force with which your body presses against the walls and ceiling increases with every inhalation, until soon the pressure becomes too great – the walls and ceiling begin to crack, and finally to disintegrate. Your body now commences to expand into infinite space.

In bringing the exercise to a close let the air out of your body in one long exhalation. This will bring your body back to its normal size, a fact of which you can convince yourself as soon as you open your eyes.

DECREASING SIZE OF BODY

Again your eyes are closed. With every forceful exhalation, feel your body become smaller. It shrinks still more each time you breathe out, continuing to shrivel until at last it is as small as a mustard seed. If your mind is distracted while you are becoming smaller – if a thought is allowed to come into the conscious mind – the effect is destroyed, and before you can open your eyes your body is again its normal size.

When your body has become as small as a mustard seed, you may breathe in deeply, and 'pump' yourself up in one prolonged inhalation, bringing yourself once more to human proportions. You could, however, continue the exercise and become smaller even than a mustard seed, until at last you would be as small as an atom, which then would be taken up in the atmosphere and freely circulated in space.

FLOATING IN THE AIR

The practitioner feels his body becoming lighter. He must focus his entire attention on this imagined feeling of decreased bodily weight, otherwise the effort will be wasted.

With constant concentration the force of gravity is gradually overcome. No longer earthbound, the body slowly begins to rise. The ceiling of the room opens, the body becomes a balloon and soars aloft into a blue sky. Carried by the winds, the student floats over peaceful valleys, winding rivers, and snow-capped mountains. Ever higher he goes, experiencing a sensation of noiseless, effortless floating.

He who can successfully practise this exercise has achieved levitation, at least where it matters most – in his own mind.

FILLING THE BODY WITH WATER

This particular exercise is practised to flush away, in a psychic sense, impurities from body and mind. With the first exhalation one feels water enter the body through whatever parts are touching the floor. With each new exhalation, the water is felt to rise higher. The body becomes a pump; as the air is expelled a vacuum is created, and more water enters. First it fills the legs, then the abdomen, the chest cavity, both arms; it rises in the neck and gradually fills the head, until finally it reaches to the top of the skull. The water is allowed to remain in the body for a while, until all physical defects and undesirable psychological qualities are dissolved in it. Finally, with a very deep inhalation the water is pressed out, taking with it all that is negative.

AWARENESS OF THE DIFFERENT PARTS
OF THE BODY

For students who are just setting out to gain control over their minds, this particular mental exercise is best practised in *savasana*.

To become aware of the different parts of the body, one directs one's whole consciousness to the selected section. If the left foot has been decided upon, one increases one's awareness of that foot to the exclusion of all other parts of the body. One tries mentally to feel not only the enveloping skin, but also the flesh and bones, and even the blood circulating through the member. When a tingling sensation is felt in the foot, one can be satisfied that the concentration has been complete. One may then continue the exercise with other parts, until the whole body has received attention.

THE LOTUS IN THE HEART

A lotus flower is visualized in the centre of the heart. It is seen as a white flower with twelve petals. At the commencement of the exercise, the face of the lotus is turned downward. With each inhalation, it is slightly raised. There is a light inside the flower, a light that gradually becomes clearer as the face of the lotus is raised higher. When finally the shining lotus is upright, the practitioner is engulfed in its radiant light.

MANTRAS

A *mantra* is, in essence, a spiritual formula. Through its constant and rhythmic repetition (*japa*), the student aims for identification with the subject of the *mantra*. If there is only concentration on the sound of the word (or words) of the *mantra*, the *japa* is merely a concentration exercise, resulting in calmness and singleness of mind. But when the *mantra* is repeated with full consideration of the meaning of the words and the ideas they embody, the exercise becomes meditation.

Mantras can be recited audibly (*vachika japa*); softly (*upanshu japa*), where there is only a whisper which others cannot hear; or silently (*manasa japa*), where neither lips nor vocal chords move, and the *japa* is in the mind only. The soft *japa* is more beneficial than the spoken one, while the silent *japa* is the most powerful of the three.

Mantras should be recited at an even tempo, not too fast and not too slowly. While chanting – be it loudly, softly, or silently – the student may use a *mala* (rosary) of one hundred and eight beads.

Om Mantra

The word *Om* (pronounced as in 'home', and sometimes transcribed as *Aum*) has from time immemorial been the highest and most revered yogic *mantra*. Its sound is held to include each of the fifty letters of the Sanskrit alphabet, and thus *Om* contains the name of everything.

There are different ways of repeating the all-inclusive *Om* *mantra*.

Om can be joined to the inflowing breath, and again to the outflowing breath, till the whole mind is filled with the sacred syllable and is vibrating with its essence.

After taking a complete breath, you can chant *Om*. Let the sound commence deep down in the throat, let it gradually move forward, and continue the prolonged, resonant vibration of the 'm' when the lips are closed. The chant should be clear and even.

If they have the opportunity, students can chant the *mantra* together, sending the powerful waves of the beautiful sound to their hearts, to one another, to all Yoga students everywhere, to teachers and adepts, and to all living beings. For added reverence they may hold the hands in front of the chest, as in prayer.

Sa'ha Mantra

As you inhale deeply through the nose, and the air flows in noisily, join the syllable *sa* to the incoming breath, making it exactly as long as that breath. When you breathe out, join the syllable *ha* to the outflowing breath, again making the syllable exactly as long as that breath. Breathing calmly and evenly, you are thus constantly repeating Sa-ha. This combination, freely translated, stands in Sanskrit for 'That I am', That indicating the Eternal. The exalted conclusion of Yoga (*Vedanta*) philosophy is that the Eternal is in everything and *is* everything. To come to the realization that you are the Eternal is the ultimate aim of your yogic training. At the present stage of your progress the conscious repetition of the beautiful *Sa'ha* *mantra* is of great benefit to you.

The *Gheranda Samhita* states (V, 84) that there are, during a day and night, twenty-one thousand six hundred such respirations (you will find this correct if you breathe in and out at a rate of fifteen times per minute). After you have practised the repetition of the *Sa'ha mantra* for a while you will hear that the incoming breath does actually sound like *sa*, and the outgoing breath like *ha*. This leads to the important realization that, during every twenty-four hour period, you are twenty-one thousand six hundred times proclaiming your divine nature. And not only you, but every living being, whether aware of it or not, constantly recites this sacred *mantra*.

Gayatri Mantra

The *Gayatri mantra*, compiled by the sage Viswamitri, has for centuries been used as a *mantra* and prayer by the members of the highest caste in India, the Brahmins. The following are the fourteen words of this *mantra*: *Om; Bhur Bhuvah Swah; Tat Savitur Varenyam; Bhargo Devasya dhimahi; Dhiyo jo nah prachodayat.*

The first nine words in the *mantra* are names of the Divine, while the word *dhimahi* signifies worship or meditation. The last sentence of the *mantra* is a prayer for enlightenment.

AWAKENING KUNDALINI

According to ancient yogi theory, *Prana,* or life-force, circulates in the body through a dense network of 72,000 *nadis,* thus activating all the organs and senses. These *nadis* can be compared to the nerve channels in the human body. All the 72,000 *nadis* spring from a centre at the base of the spine. The principal *nadi* is called *sushumna.* It runs inside the spinal column and through the brain to the crown of the head. The *Prana* that flows through the *sushumna* is in the form of the goddess Kundalini. Normally Kundalini is asleep in her cave (*kanda*) at the base of the spine.

The goddess is described as a snake, lying curled up in three and one-half coils. With her mouth, she closes off the lower entrance of the fine *sushumna* channel.

The aim of Kundalini Yoga, also called Laya Yoga, is to awaken Kundalini, so that she stirs, hisses, and commences to move up through the *sushumna* channel in a journey to the top of the head where the Lord Shiva, third god of the Hindu trinity, abides. Shiva represents pure consciousness, and Kundalini is a power of *Shakti*. The object of Kundalini Yoga is achieved when the union of Shiva and Shakti takes place.

Deep concentration and meditation are required in order to rouse Kundalini and to clear the road for her upward journey, for the *sushumna* channel is blocked by the first six of seven major centres, or *chakras,* which are threaded upon the principal *nadi.* The student intent on making use of the profound mental exercise provided by the actual practice of Kundalini Yoga, should learn all he can about the seven *chakras,* so that he can find them in introspective exploration, and through his mind's eye visualize the centres in their respective places. By unmovingly holding all his mental faculties in the *chakras,* he will be able to unlock them, thus clearing the way for Kundalini. First the *muladhara chakra* at the lower aperture of the *sushumna* is opened; once the she-serpent nas entered the *sushumna* of her own accord, she is taken from *chakra* to *chakra;* as the centres are unlocked, Kundalini continues her upward journey towards her spiritual spouse, the Lord Shiva, residing in the seventh and highest *chakra,* the *sahasrara chakra.*

Muladhara Chakra

This *chakra* is situated at the base of the spinal column, between the genital organs and the anus. It is represented by a yellow lotus with four crimson petals and is associated with the element earth and the sense of smell.

Its basic *bija,* or seed sound, is *lam.* The vowel in *lam* is kept short and pronounced as in the word 'run'. (The vowels of the *bijas* of the following four *chakras* are pronounced exactly the same.) The last consonant, the 'm' is continued evenly with the lips closed for as long as the supply of air lasts.

While meditating upon a chakra, the student can, for quicker results, chant its *bija,* the vibrations of which help to open each particular *chakra.*

Svadhisthana Chakra

Situated at the root of the penis, the *svadhisthana chakra* is represented by a white lotus with six vermilion petals. It is allied with the element water and the sense of taste.

Its *bija mantra* (seed sound) is *vam.*

Manipura Chakra

In the *sushumna,* at the height of the navel, is the *manipura chakra.* It is depicted as a red lotus with ten golden petals. It is linked with the element fire and the sense of sight.

The *bija mantra* of this *chakra* is *ram.*

Anahata Chakra

The *anahata chakra,* in the region of the heart, is represented by a grey lotus with twelve flaming red petals. The associated element and sense are air and touch, respectively.

Its *bija mantra* is *yam.*

Vishuddha Chakra

Situated in the throat region, directly beneath the larynx, the *vishuddha chakra* is depicted as a white lotus with sixteen purple petals. It is allied with the element ether and the sense of hearing.

The *bija mantra* of this *chakra* is *ham.*

Ajna Chakra

The *ajna chakra* is the command centre, situated midway between the eyebrows. It governs and unifies the faculties represented in the foregoing five *chakras*. The *ajna chakra* is the *chakra* of the mind, and it is represented by a brilliant white lotus with two white petals.

The *bija mantra* of the mind centre is *Om,* and it is in this centre that the yogi recites *Om* at the time of departure from his physical garb.

Sahasrara Chakra

At the crown of the head, shining with the brilliance of many suns, is the thousand-petalled lotus, the *sahasrara chakra*. It is the seat of pure consciousness, represented by Shiva.

As a preliminary exercise to concentration and meditation upon the *chakras,* yogic breathing is practised. This has the effect of purifying the *nadis* and paves the way for opening the *chakras*.

Kundalini is awakened by meditation upon her as she lies in her resting place, and this meditation can, according to the *Gheranda Samhita* (III, 82), be accompanied by frequently contracting and relaxing the anus. A further technique called *Shakticalana,* which means 'moving Shakti', is employed to make Kundalini enter the *sushumna* channel. *Shakticalana* is performed by inhaling deeply, and, while holding the breath, slowly contracting the anus so that the excretory energy (*apana*) is forced upward [*Gheranda Samhita* (III, 54, 55)]. Similar instructions are given in the *Hatha Yoga Pradipika* (I, 48), which also states (III, 29) that results can be obtained by repeatedly bumping the buttocks on the floor in a gentle manner.

The destination of Shakti (Kundalini) is the *sahasrara chakra,* where union with Shiva takes place – a union symbolic of the joining of man's latent energy with pure consciousness. At the finish of the yogi's meditation, Shakti, pregnant with knowledge, retreats to her resting place at the base of the spine. As she goes downward, she vitalizes the *chakras,* endowing them with consciousness and power. Eventually the *chakras* wiil remain open permanently, leaving a free passage for pure consciousness to flow through.

CONCENTRATION ON COMMAND CENTRE

Because of its position in the subcortical area of the brain, midway between the eyebrows, and because of the importance of its functions from a yogic point of view, the *ajna chakra,* or command centre, provides an excellent subject for concentration.

The student should close his eyes as he brings the full attention of his mind to the point between the eyebrows. His concentration will be deep if he unintentionally holds his breath. In the beginning it may help the unruly mind if the closed eyes 'look up' to the spot where the mind is to be focused, but this should not be done to such an extent, and for such a duration, that discomfort is felt.

Stimulation of this centre through intense and unmoving concentration will give the practitioner greater mental powers.

BINDU MANIPULATION

An advanced mental exercise is provided by *bindu* manipulation. *Bindu* means point, or dot.

As a first stage, the *bindu* has to be visualized in the command centre between the eyebrows. The *bindu* can be seen in the form of a tiny transparent pearl. This part of the exercise has to be continued until the vision becomes absolutely clear.

Manipulation of the *bindu* means that it is moved up from the *ajna chakra* to the *sahasrara chakra,* in the cortical area of the physical brain, at the crown of the head. The tiny pearl is to be regarded as containing the essence of the mind, which will be further enriched when brought into direct contact with the consciousness in the high *sahasrara chakra.*

During slow and even inhalation, the attention of the mind is unfalteringly held on the *bindu,* which is made to move up through a nerve channel (the *sushumna nadi*) to the *sahasrara* centre. For the duration of the breath retention the *bindu* remains in the *sahasrara chakra,* where it is charged with the pure consciousness present there. As the breath is let out, almost imperceptibly, the now brilliant pearl is carefully guided back through the *sushumna nadi* to the *ajna chakra*, which it fills with effulgent light.

The exercise is completed by prolonged meditation in the radiant *ajna chakra*.

NADA BANDHA

As in the Hatha and Laya branches of Yoga certain muscular locks, or *bandhas,* are applied, so in the science of Raja Yoga a mental lock can be practised. This psychological lock is called *nada bandha. Nada* means sound, especially internal sound, and in *nada bandha* the practitioner listens with the 'inner' ear to the sound of the Supreme. The whole universe is in vibration – the vibration of the Infinite – and this omnipresent divine music is, on a superphysical plane, manifested in the individual as a singing sound in the head.

In performing *nada bandha,* the practitioner focuses all his mental faculties within the *ajna chakra,* the subtle centre midway between the eyebrows. There, with all his psychic energy, he tunes in to perceive the music of the *Supreme,* which is *Om.*

CHAPTER SIX

Yogic Discipline
in Daily Life

To attain the highest in Yoga, one's whole life should be directed towards that goal. Every deed performed and every thought entertained should be compatible with the yogic teachings. One may practise diligently for two hours each day in the solitude of a quiet room – and this would be wonderful – but one still must carry one's convictions into daily life and live according to them in order to achieve ultimate success.

The Yoga student should fulfil his worldly duties to the best of his abilities, happy to be of service to others. His work should not be done purely for financial reward or other selfish interests. Instead of thinking about personal gain, he should think of the good of his fellow man. To serve man is to serve the Divine.

The student will find many opportunities in everyday life to practise concentration, to exercise self-control, to improve his willpower, and to act selflessly. Concentrating on everything that he does, he aims for perfection in whatever he undertakes. In performing a particular action, he is fully aware of what he is doing. Inefficiency is a thing of the past. He overcomes his dislikes by singling out work he previously avoided. Now he purposely concentrates upon it, and finds pleasure in acquitting himself of such obligations.

Difficulties, no matter in what form or degree, provide the student with welcome challenges. Great difficulties have been overcome by many people in the past, and will be overcome in the future. In proving himself a master of every situation, the student will be a shining example to others.

Whatever happens, the student should try to remain calm.

He should attempt to maintain his mental equilibrium in all circumstances. A calm mind is a great friend. If one becomes excited, or even angry, matters are likely to become more complicated, and troubles may pile up. A philosophical attitude is best. If something seemingly adverse happens, one should not think of it as such. Whether a thing or occurrence seems adverse depends on one's attitude towards it. In the face of apparent adversity, one should try to retain not only an outward air of calmness but also, and even more determinedly, one should be intent on maintaining one's inward composure. Great mental strength will be the result of continual practice in preserving a peaceful state of mind.

The Yoga student should pay attention to what he says. Spoken words are but manifestations of inner thoughts. As a first step, the student should relinquish all talk about selfish desires, and of everything else that is detrimental to success in Yoga. As a last step, he should relinquish all adverse thoughts. In conversation he should try to stick to the subject under discussion. This is a form of concentration, and it is interesting to discover how difficult many people find it. Instead of wasting his own efforts, and other people's time, the Yoga student aims to be concise and correct in every thought he utters. He tries to cover the important aspects of whatever subject is being discussed, and he applies the same discipline to his thinking. His mind should not be cluttered with trivialities. Because the student learns to understand himself, and through this other people, he does not utter a word about others that is critical or negative. As he progresses in Yoga, his understanding will deepen, and critical thoughts will turn into brotherly love. The student will truly feel 'malice toward none, and charity for all'. Such an attitude will create a harmonious atmosphere in the world as well as in the practitioner's mind.

The serious student does not engage in futile discussion, nor does he become involved in argument. He is convinced of the rightness of his ways, and quietly, yet firmly, he continues his training. He never boasts to others about his mental achievements. He speaks less, and if circumstances allow, he may even enter a period of complete silence, or *mouna*. He becomes a real *mouni* when he is not only outwardly silent, but when his mind also is quiet and undisturbed.

Self-restraint is to be practised at all times, and negative habits are to be overcome. A great measure of willpower will often be required, but this is a joy to the Yoga student. He likes to exercise his willpower, which can only become stronger through practice. Opportunities abound in which he can test and sharpen this faculty, which otherwise may fade if not regularly used. First, bad habits are shaken off as the snake casts off its old skin. High priority should be given to the elimination of smoking and the drinking of alcohol. These habits are enslaving, and the Yoga student does not want to be dominated by any such things. Furthermore, such addictions are injurious to bodily health. Smoking affects the lungs, while alcohol befouls the bloodstream and befogs the mind. A little alcohol will not harm the student, but first he should completely overcome any need for it; that he has indeed mastered his weakness can be proven by a prolonged period of abstinence from alcoholic beverages. Afterwards he will be able to say no to a drink at any time.

Desire for objects is developed almost from birth. A rattle is temptingly shaken in front of a baby's eyes, the young child's desires are awakened, and he grabs for the toy. This pattern is continued through life. We are seduced by shiny things, and want to call them ours. Once we have them, often we no longer appreciate them and carelessly discard them, much as the baby throws its newly-acquired rattle out of its crib. These reflections should not result in a disgust for objects. Things themselves are neither good nor bad; it is only one's mental attitude towards them that makes them seem so. Both aversion and attachment should be overcome equally.

The desire for objects keeps the mind in a continuous state of turmoil, ever thinking of more things to be gotten. It is this feverish mental state that the Raja Yoga student seeks to fight by the practice of inward non-attachment. Being surrounded by temptations makes his battle an even more interesting one. He girds for the contest and sets out to annihilate the distracting influences which are so deeply rooted in his lower mind. The fight must be a relentless one because the enemy is powerful. Sensual desires will raise their heads again as soon as the struggle is eased. Living on the bare necessities of life for a time will be of great help to the student.

The student should learn to rely only on himself. Dependence

on others must be overcome, along with the need for appreciation and praise. The student will find an abundance of strength
and inspiration from his study and practice of the yogic teachings. He no longer will need to rely on other people. He will
become an exemplary tower of independent strength.

Fasting, albeit in moderation, provides another avenue for
the practice of willpower. Extreme fasts, however, are dis-
approved, as is clearly explained in the often cited verse (VI, 16)
of the *Bhagavad Gita*; but an excessive intake of food is certainly
to be curbed. Of course a certain amount of food is essential
for maintaining bodily health, but this quantity is much smaller
than some people think. As mental training, the extravagant
craving for food can be subdued by setting aside one day a
week in which no food is taken at all, and only water is drunk.
This practice will also help to cleanse the system, but it should
not be adopted by people who are under-weight. A mild yet
very beneficial form of overcoming the craving for food is to
eat very slowly.

The yogic regime of life also includes abstinence from sex.
For the student intent on complete mastery over his mind, it
is imperative that he learn to control the sexual urge. He does
not want to be a slave to his sexual passions, just as he does
not want to be a weakling in regard to any other desires. Sex
does not have to be given up forever, but the desire for it must
be brought under control. How does the student go about it?
The most drastic method is to relinquish all sexual activity, and
all thoughts on the subject. The company of lustful members of
the opposite sex is avoided, and all thoughts of sex are suppressed
by the substitution of totally different thoughts.

Some people find it easier than others to practise abstinence
from sex. The sexual urge is not felt with the same intensity
by all; lack of opportunity or abundance of it also plays a
significant role. If the student is a happily married man, enjoying a harmonious sex life, it cannot be expected that he will
suddenly give up that which brings him and his partner so close
together. There is, furthermore, the necessity of sex for procreation. If everyone were to give up sex altogether, it would
after all, mean the rather abrupt end of the human race. The
student living in partnership practises moderation. If both the
man and the woman are students of mental Yoga, then tem

porary abstention can provide a worthwhile challenge.

On the subject of sex, conflicting opinions are given in yogic literature. On the one hand, the aspirant of Yoga is bidden to maintain the strictest continence in deed and thought, while on the other different meanings behind the sexual act are propounded. Thus a case is made for actual participation in *maithuna,* or sexual union, for specified purposes. *Maithuna* is lifted onto a spiritual plane when the participants regard themselves as actors in a divine play. Also, in various places, techniques are described that may be practised during *maithuna* for the attainment of self-control and the gaining of strength. The *sukra,* or semen, was regarded by the ancients as containing the essence of man, and therefore preventing its loss would mean preserving one's strength. Coitus is prolonged, and under the stimulus of excitement, more seminal fluid is produced. Ejaculation should not take place, and to stop the 'shooting of the seed', a *mudra,* or lock, is applied, such as the *khecari mudra,* in which the tongue is folded back and made to reach for the throat. Thought remains motionless, and the *sukra* is not emitted, not even in 'the embrace of a young and passionate woman'. After self-control is thus established, the modern student should allow orgasm to take place, as the incomplete sexual act will cause congestion in the sexual organs, and this may cause pain.

In religious rites sexual intercourse was seen as a symbolic act. Woman became a consecrated place for the performance of a sacrifice. Her lap was the altar in which burnt the sacrificial fire, and therein the devotee made his offering. Before the act considerable time was spent in meditation on its symbolic meaning. *Maithuna* thus performed with purified mind can only make a basic instinct sublime.

The play of cosmic forces, too, can be seen at work in the copulating human couple, passionately striving for oneness. The fertile woman is regarded as the representative of all the female aspects of nature, while the powerful man represents all male aspects. Orgasm becomes a mystical experience. Similarly, the ecstatic union of the human couple is seen as the mystic union of matter and spirit, in which the woman is seen as an incarnation of *prakriti,* or matter, and her partner as an incarnation of *purusha,* or spirit. In *maithuna* the male remains static, as the immovable spirit, while all activity comes from the side of his female counterpart, representing active matter.

The student of mental Yoga may decide for himself to which school he rightly belongs, and which approach is best suited to his particular case. Reflection on the subject, together with the study of Yoga philosophy, will enable him to see sex in a different light. Instead of disturbing his mind sex will become a surpassingly sublime experience. But before he decides what is good for him he should, if he has the opportunity, sincerely practise continence for a period. Not only should he refrain from the actual deed during that time, but he should also attempt to ban all thoughts of it from his mind. He should regard members of the opposite sex as spiritual beings living in physical bodies. Once he feels he has mastered his sexual desires to a sufficient degree, he may again participate in a moderate sex life.

CHAPTER SEVEN

Meditation

The purpose of yogic meditation is to awaken one's higher consciousness. Through the various meditative practices, the meditator aspires to attune himself to the spiritual principle within his being. In deep meditation the mind is transcended, and a new dimension of existence is entered.

The mind is the connecting link between the body and the spirit. For some, the mind is closely tied to bodily needs and passions; for others, the mind is more congruent with spiritual values. All previous yogic training has been undertaken in order to banish the first mentioned condition, and to bring about the latter. Meditation will now accelerate this process.

The Yoga teachings suggest that the human mind can be seen as divided into three regions, which can be termed the subconscious mind, the conscious mind, and the superconscious mind. Basic instincts and egotistical desires are the properties of the subconscious mind, where man is closest to the animal; the conscious mind is the seat of reason and intellect, and deals with everyday living; the superconscious mind is that region of the mind that is closest to the self – the spark of Infinity in man – and it is the source of all that is good in human nature. Lofty aspirations and noble thoughts, unselfish love and affection for humanity, ethical principles and inspiring ideas – all spring from that realm of the mind that lies above ordinary consciousness.

Man, as we generally know him, is an unfinished product. However, he possesses within himself the possibility of spiritual evolution, and, through his own efforts, he can elevate himself to the plane of the superconscious mind.

Meditation can be undertaken successfully only after the art of concentration has been mastered, and thought and feeling have been brought under control. Once meditation is begun, it is best practised every day, under conditions similar to those required for exercises in concentration. Worldly duties should not be neglected; on the other hand, the affairs of the world should not be allowed to take up all of one's time and devotion, at least not at this stage. According to one's inclination, one may practise meditation directly after one has done some yogic breathing and concentration, for these exercises will prepare the mind. Provided one is advanced enough, one may commence meditation at once and continue for the whole of the period set aside each day for this purpose.

Yogic meditation differs from normal concentration. Whereas in concentration the subject can be either a concrete object or an abstract idea, in meditation the subject is always of a spiritual nature. The techniques applied may also differ. For one thing, in meditation there must be no noticeable effort at all. The mind has been subjected to a profound training programme and can now be held in check for prolonged periods. External and internal distractions no longer pose a threat during meditation practice.

The thought or idea to be pondered is carefully selected and then held in the mind for some time. After this there may be two further developments. In the first method, the meditator explores various aspects of the central theme, paying equal attention to each angle. Finally, all the aspects in their entirety are projected onto the mental screen. In the second method, the central theme is momentarily dropped from the field of consciousness; while the meditator holds his mind still, he waits for associated ideas to come into his awareness. Everything that is relative to the subject under consideration is allowed into the mind, reflected upon, and subsequently dismissed to make room for the next thought. At the end of the meditation the central theme is re-introduced, and will then be seen in depth.

Thoughts to be used as subjects for meditation can be found

in abundance in the *Upanishads* and the *Bhagavad Gita* (see Chapters X and XI, respectively, of this book). The meditator selects a quotation that strikes him as suitable, and then reflects upon its meaning. Turning the passage over in his mind, he endeavours to extract its spiritual message.

MEDITATION ON OM

Om: such a short syllable, and yet it is used to indicate all that is in and beyond the Universe. Maker, Sustainer, and Transformer of the Cosmos; the most abstract aspect of Divinity; and the sounds and vibrations of every manifestation – all are denoted by this monosyllabic *mantra*. When the Hindu gasps *Om* in his dying moments, his soul is liberated.

Realizing the profound meaning of the *mantra,* the meditator reverently lets *Om* resound in his mind until at last the sacred vibration begins to permeate his whole being. Meditating on *Om* with such intensity will help in achieving spiritual aims. *Om* is the bow, the mind is the arrow, and Supreme Reality is the target.

MEDITATION ON ONENESS

The student here makes oneness the subject of his meditation. Yoga teaches that everything that exists is a manifestation of the one Divine Life. This means that there is a relationship between all that moves and breathes. First the student may reflect upon the points of resemblance between his blood relations and himself. Next he may seek out similarities among all the people he knows. He may widen his inquiry and dwell upon the things he has in common with his countrymen. Ignoring artificial borders and prejudices, he next includes people of various races in his quest for corresponding essentials. Having seen the unity of the human race, he widens his horizon still further, examining the common factors among all living creatures, be they plant, animal, or man.

Realizing the oneness of life and his relationship to all life, the student concludes his meditation by sending a deeply felt message of all-embracing love to all that lives.

WHAT AM I?

In this meditation each person silently but earnestly asks himself the question 'What am I?' We all sense that we are 'something', but we are either ignorant of, or vague about, what this 'something' might be. In order to find our essence, we let the different aspects of our being parade one by one through our minds, subjecting each to a thorough analysis. We are not the person that strangers may think us, for we show our friends a different face. Society has compelled us to develop certain characteristics which are no part of our true personality, and which we use merely as a facade for everyday living, as well as for protection. A man usually presents himself to his supervisor in a different manner from that in which he appears to those whom he himself supervises. Business acquaintances do not know him as his wife knows him. His children see him in a different light from that in which his parents view him. So he is not what the world in general thinks him to be.

Are we no more than our bodies? Scientists tell us that man's body undergoes complete renewal during the course of seven years. Therefore, we cannot be the body, for even though the body changes – and we can notice the change – we feel that we are still one and the same being. The things that happened to us in childhood happened to the same person who is now the adult.

Are we identical with our faculty of thought? No, because we can observe the thinking process; thoughts come and go, and we are more than those transient thoughts. We are also not identical with our intellect and our capacity for reasoning, for we can use both as our instruments. Likewise, our emotions may be fickle or deeply felt, but even the latter tend to disappear with the passing of time. As a man can speak of 'my coat' and 'my car,' so he can say 'my body,' 'my intellect,' and 'my feeling'. He speaks of those things and faculties as belonging to him and as being part of him, but he does not think himself to be identical with them, any more than he identifies himself with his possessions.

Man knows intuitively that he is more than his changing body, more than his intellect, more than his fleeting thoughts, and more than his fluctuating emotions. He senses that there is something deep within his personality that remains constant even through the passage of time and amidst successive changes. As he analyses himself, he rejects aspect after aspect, until finally he is left with the notion 'I'. This sense of self cannot be reasoned away. Throughout his life, the feeling 'I' will remain the same. It is this 'I' to which everything happens, and which feels, speaks, and acts. The 'I' feeling persists even in dreams. It remains constant throughout man's physical and mental development, from early infancy to mature adulthood. It is the one permanent feature of his being, and when all his actions are analysed, it is found that 'I' is man's chief concern; 'I' is foremost in his thoughts and considerations, everything pivots around this central thought 'I'. No matter what happens, man always feels this 'I'.

At the conclusion of the meditation entitled 'What am I?' the meditator asks himself from whence this consciousness of himself springs.

I AM

In this meditation the student does not concern himself with any intellectual concept of what he is, or what he is not, but solely with the fact that he *is*. Concentrating fully, first slowly and then deliberately he repeats several times to himself the sentence 'I Am'. Then the thought process is arrested and the practitioner meditates upon the idea embodied in this short but significant sentence. He endeavours to feel with intense awareness the fact that he *is*. During the course of the meditation, the student may from time to time repeat the central theme 'I Am'. After each mental utterance he plunges with renewed vigour into the intense feeling of existence.

SUPRA-MENTAL MEDITATION

In the meditation techniques described earlier, there was always a central thought or idea that was used as subject or starting point of the meditation. In supra-mental meditation there is no such theme. The thought process is not brought into play at all. The mind is kept perfectly still. Because thought-free meditation is very difficult, it is advisable that the other techniques be mastered first.

For successful supra-mental meditation it is essential that the mind be held still for a prolonged period; this can be accomplished only after long and intensive practice. Keeping thoughts out of the mind should require no noticeable effort whatsoever. When thought is ejected from the mind, only consciousness remains.

Although the meditator's mind is devoid of all activity, he is extremely alert. As he dwells on inner peace, his mind becomes extremely sensitive and receptive. It is in such moments of deep tranquillity that man receives the loftiest of revelations. From the mystic stillness arise the supreme manifestations of That, which are *Sat, Chit, Ananda*—Being, Consciousness, Bliss. Slowly they begin to filter through the silence. A higher consciousness is dawning, and the attainment of the ultimate yogic goal – the blissful state of *samadhi* – is near.

CHAPTER EIGHT

Samadhi

The attainment of the state of *samadhi* is the crowning fulfilment of a long yogic training programme. As a result of his spiritual efforts, the meditator becomes acutely aware of the Divine Principle within his being. In *samadhi* the meditator transcends the limitations of the mind and experiences the Being, Consciousness, and Bliss of That which alone *is*.

In order to attain *samadhi* all preconceived notions about the self are to be dropped from the mind. Intellectual concepts and abstract ideas must be discarded. Divinity is beyond the province of the intellect. The borders of the spiritual realm can be reached by intellectual inquiry, but the faculty for thinking and reasoning can take one no further. The superconscious state is only attained in supra-mental meditation. Such thought-free contemplation is preceded by a meditation of the kind which in the past has given the practitioner a sensation of utmost serenity, making him feel as if he were lifted above the normal state of consciousness. The advanced meditator knows for himself how he brought about such a condition. He may have dwelt extensively upon the thought that his nature is divine. 'I am, in essence, a divine spirit' may have been his frequent and deliberate repetition. He may have silently affirmed to himself that he is an indestructible and imperishable part of the One Life. Any aspect of the Supreme Being may have been the subject of his meditation.

Samadhi takes place on the superconscious plane. As such it is an experience that is not communicable by mere words.

Modes of expression primarily devised to denote happenings on the physical and mental planes become inadequate when those planes are left behind. Verbalizing, metaphorical or otherwise, can give no more than an indication of what occurs during a supersensual event.

Sitting perfectly still, his body forgotten and his mind held unwaveringly in passive purity, the yogi is engulfed by an intense and joyous feeling of exaltation. The spark of divinity within him leaps into a lustrous flame. The yogi experiences boundless Being, infinite Consciousness, and Ecstatic Bliss in one sublime sensation. His limited personality expands into unlimited Being. He is aware of omnipresent Consciousness. All discords are utterly dissolved in an uplifting transport of all-embracing Bliss. Dualities do not exist in the radiant realm of the Self. It is an eternal world of transcendental joy and ineffable peace. How can words ever suffice to describe That which is indescribable?

When the timeless moment of spiritual illumination subsides, the yogi is left a changed man. The world as viewed through the eyes of ordinary human beings seems to him unreal. A transformation has taken place in his mind. His former personality has been annihilated. After dwelling on the pinnacle of Supreme Bliss in ecstatic union with Divine Self, the yogi finds that all egotistical thoughts and desires, or remnants thereof, have been destroyed, and in their place has come lasting non-attachment.

CHAPTER NINE

India's
Sacred Heritage

For the student intent on understanding Indian religion and philosophy, it is essential that he knows something of the *Vedas,* and that he realizes their overwhelming importance and influence.

The word *veda* means knowledge – specifically, spiritual knowledge. What we now know as the *Vedas* is a vast body of material which began to grow into its present form thousands of years ago, over a period of many centuries. The sacred heritage was handed down orally from teacher to disciple, through the devotion of countless adherents, from one generation to another.

The *Vedas* are made up of the utterances of ancient poets, priests, and forest saints, or *rishis* (seers), in the form of chants, prayers, formulas for sacrifices, magic, and rituals, and discussions on the meaning and the nature of Supreme Reality.

The *Vedas* are the oldest literary compositions in any Indo-Aryan language. They have their roots in the legendary prehistoric times. Professor Max Müller (1823-1900), an eminent scholar and pioneer who devoted a lifetime to the study and translation of India's classic books, came to the conclusion that the *Vedas* were completed before 600 B.C. He decided that the whole of Verdic literature must have existed before the rise of Buddhism, since the teachings of Buddha, born in 563 B.C., were based largely on the *Upanishads,* the philosophical and final sections of the *Vedas.*

The *Vedas* are divided into four books: the *Rig Veda,* the

Yajur Veda, the *Sama Veda,* and the *Atharva Veda.* This four-fold division is attributed to the sage Vyasa, who is thought to have lived about 500 B.C. The *Rig Veda* is the first and largest of the four books; *rig* means 'verse', and the *Rig Veda* is mostly a collection of hymns of praise and prayer to a variety of deities In *Yajur Veda,* besides verses from the *Rig Veda,* are found many sacrificial prayers. The *Sama Veda,* or *Veda of Melodies* also contains chants taken from the *Rig Veda.* The *Atharva Veda* is primarily a collection of hymns and spells.

Each *Veda* also contains exalted spiritual truths – the teachings of sages who renounced the world, retired to the forests and there spent many years in profound contemplation. Their wisdom is collected in the *Upanishads,* which form the concluding part of each *Veda.*

In 1856 English engineers who were engaged in the construction of the East Indian Railway from Karachi to Lahore considered themselves lucky that the line they were building ran close to the ruins of two ancient cities, one along the southern end of the line, the other along the northern end. In the ruins of these cities they discovered an abundance of fine bricks which solved the problem of finding ballast for the railway line. The engineers and workmen made good use of this ready supply of building materials, little realizing the antiquity and importance of their find, nor anticipating the wrath they would incur from later researchers. While collecting bricks, the workmen found several antiquities which aroused the curiosity of people interested in India's history. However, quite some time elapsed before any definite measures were taken. Finally archaeologists began to conduct excavation work at the sites. Their efforts revealed the existence of a great prehistoric empire in north-western India, which became known as the Harappa, or Indus Valley, Civilization. One of the ancient cities was Harappa, situated in the Punjab on the left bank of the river Ravi, about one hundred miles southwest of Lahore. The other city was Mahenjo-daro in Sind, built on the right bank of the river Indus, and situated about two hundred miles north of Karachi.

Excavation work on the Harappa site commenced in 1920 and on the Mohenjo-daro site in 1922. It soon became evident that the two cities had been the twin capitals of an empire that had enjoyed an apparently uninterrupted, nearly static existence for about a thousand years, the period estimated to be from approximately 2500 B.C. to 1500 B.C. Some three hundred and fifty miles apart, the cities were connected by navigable rivers – the Ravi being a tributary of the Indus – and showed striking similarities. They were laid out to a common ground plan, and each had a surface of about one square mile; each had a defence citadel towering over the other buildings; the size of the bricks used in both cities was uniform, as was the size of the bricks used in constructing the towns and villages around and between the two major cities.

The people of the Harappa civilization were of mixed race, although the Mediterranean type was probably predominant. Occupied in agriculture, they grew wheat, barley and cotton. Their domesticated animals included humped bulls, buffaloes, goats, sheep, and pigs. They knew how to forge and cast copper and bronze for the manufacture of simple tools and weapons, and they were well advanced in the making of pottery. Although their script has not as yet been deciphered, they had developed the art of writing.

Very little is known about the religious beliefs of these pre-historic people. It is thought that they were worshippers of a mother goddess; a seal has been found showing a female from whose womb a plant sprouts forth. She probably represented a goddess of earth and vegetation, and her male consort could have been a prototype of the god Shiva, since among the steatite stamp-seals found was one engraved with the figure of a horned, three-faced male deity. This possible forerunner of Shiva was seated in a yogic posture; legs bent, feet heel-to-heel. His eyes were focused on the tip of the nose, and he was surrounded by four beasts – a buffalo, a rhinoceros, a tiger, and an elephant. (All four animals inhabited those regions in ancient times, but except for the tiger, no wild species have survived.)

The apparent peace of a thousand years was broken by the arrival in the region of an alien and most barbaric race, thought to have come from the west. These people called themselves *Aryan,* meaning 'noble man' in Sanskrit, an Indo-European language that was the formal tongue of the Aryan warriors, chieftains, and priests. The year 1500 B.C. is traditionally accepted as the approximate time these tribes invaded the land

of the Harappa empire. Fierce warriors, they brought swift
horse-drawn chariots onto the battlefield, and invoked the assistance and blessing of their heroic war god, Indra. The coming of
the Aryans coincides with, and was probably responsible for
the collapse of the Harappa empire.

The religious beliefs of the Aryans are expressed in the early
verses of the *Rig Veda*. They worshipped a pantheon of male
deities – such as Surya (the Sun), Agni (Fire), and Varuna (the
Sky) – which are either the powers of nature personified, or the
ideal Aryan magnified to godlike proportions. Of all their gods
the strong-armed, tawny-bearded Indra is, significantly, the
most important. About a quarter of the 1,017 hymns of the
Rig Veda are addressed to Indra, the winner of booty in battle
who may either wield a thunderbolt, or fight ferociously with
bow and arrow from his chariot. Indra is not only great in
strength, but also in size. He eats ravenously and imbibes great
quantities of soma, an intoxicating beverage derived from the
soma plant. This he drinks by the pailful – thirty lakes at a
sitting.

> On him all men must call amid the battle;
> He, high-adored, alone has power to succour.
> The man who offers him his prayers, libations,
> Him Indra's arm helps forward in his goings.
>
> They cry aloud to him amid the contest,
> Rushing to deadly combat, to protect them,
> When friend and foe lay down their lives in warfare,
> In strife to conquer peace for child and grandchild.
>
> They gird themselves, O Mighty, for the conflict,
> Provoking each the other to the quarrel;
> And when the hostile armies stand opposing,
> Then each would have great Indra for his ally.
>
> Then their obligations all they bring to Indra,
> And freely then the meats and cakes are offered;
> Then they who grudged before come rich with soma –
> Yea, they resolve to sacrifice a bullock.
>
> Yet still the god gives him success who truly,
> With willing mind pours out the draught he longs for,
> With his whole heart, nor feels regret in giving;
> To him great Indra joins himself in battle.

(IV, 24, 2–6)

Second in importance to Indra is Agni, the god of fire. Over 200 hymns are addressed to him. Originating in the clouds, he first came down to earth in the form of lightning and then went into hiding. Agni can be evoked by rubbing two sticks together. He lies concealed in the softer wood, as in a chamber. Called forth by the rubbing in the early morning hour, he suddenly emerges in gleaming brightness. The sacrificer places him on the wood; Agni greedily stretches out his sharp tongue and devours it. When the priests pour melted butter on him, he leaps up crackling and neighing, like a horse.

> All-searching is his beam, the gleaming of his light,
> His, the all-beautiful, of beauteous face and glance,
> The changing shimmer like that floats upon the stream,
> So Agni's rays gleam ever bright and never cease.
>
> (I, 143, 3)

Varuna, god of the sky, is the most sublime of the Vedic deities.

Sing a hymn, pleasing to Varuna the King – to him who spread out the earth as the butcher lays out the steer's hide in the sun.

He sent cool breezes through the woods, put mettle in the sun, rain in the clouds, wisdom in the heart, lightning in the clouds, placed the sun in the heavens, the soma plant in the mountains.

He upset the cloud-barrel and let its waters flow on heaven, air, and earth, wetting the ground and the crops.

He wets both earth and heaven, and as soon as he wishes for those clouds' water, the mountains are wrapped in thunderclouds, and the strongest walkers are tired.

(V, 85)

> His works bear witness to his might and wisdom,
> Who fashioned firm supports for earth and heaven,
> Who set on high the firmament uplifted,
> And fixed the stars and spread out earth's expanses.
>
> (VII, 86, 1)

> He mingled with the clouds his cooling breezes,
> He gave the cow her milk, the horse his spirit,
> Put wisdom in the heart, in clouds the lightning,
> The sun in heaven, on the rocks the soma.
>
> (V, 85, 2)

The sun's sure courses Varuna appointed,
He sent the streaming waters flowing onward,
The mighty path of days he first created,
And rules them as the riders guide their horses.

(VII, 87, 1)

Before the excavations and subsequent discoveries at Harappa
and Mohenjo-daro, it was generally assumed that the whole
Vedic heritage was of pure Aryan origin. But today scholars
accept it as reasonable that a merging took place – a merging
not only of race, but also of religion and philosophy. When
the Aryans settled in the newly-conquered lands, they must
have absorbed some of the native beliefs just as the people of the
Harappa civilization must have adopted certain of the Aryan
doctrines.

Now followed what is called the 'Vedic Age' – from 1500
B.C. to 600 B.C. – when the *Vedas* and the expositions contained
therein grew to maturity. In the early hymns of the *Rig Veda*
the oldest of the *Vedas*, we can see a 'primitive religion', gradually developing into something more. In the *Vedas* as a whole
we are allowed a view of human thought groping its way from
obscure darkness to the very summits of wisdom. We witness the
awakening of man's questing spirit as he expresses a sense of
wonder at the phenomena of nature. Inquiring about the all
important sun moving freely through the heavens, he asks
'Unpropped beneath, not fastened firm, how comes it, that
downward turned, he falls not down? The guide of his
ascending path – who saw it?' (IV, 13, 5).

Monotheism evolved from polytheism. Before the collection of
the hymns of the *Rig Veda* was complete, there had developed
a belief in one Being, neither male nor female, a Being raised
high above all the conditions and limitations of personality and
of human nature, the One and nevertheless the same Being that
had been referred to by such names as Indra, Agni, Varuna
Prajapati. This is evident in the song to the unknown
god:

In the beginning there arose the Golden Child [Hiranya-Garbha]
as soon as born, he alone was the lord of all that is. He established
the earth and this heaven – who is the God to whom we shall
offer sacrifice?

He who gives breath, he who gives strength, whose commands all the bright gods revere, whose shadow is immortality, whose shadow is death – who is the God to whom we shall offer sacrifice?

He who through his might became sole king of the breathing and twinkling world, who governs all this, man and beast – who is the God to whom we shall offer sacrifice?

He through whose might these snowy mountains are, and the sea, they say, with the distant river [the Rasa], he of whom these regions are indeed the two arms – who is the God to whom we shall offer sacrifice?

He through whom the awful heaven and the earth were made fast, he through whom the ether was established, and the firmament; he who measured the air in the sky – who is the God to whom we shall offer sacrifice?

He to whom heaven and earth, standing firm by his will, look up, trembling in their mind; he over whom the risen sun shines forth – who is the God to whom we shall offer sacrifice?

When the great waters went everywhere, holding the germ [*Hiranya-Garbha*], and generating light, then there arose from them the life-breath of the gods – who is the God to whom we shall offer sacrifice?

He who by his might looked even over the waters which held power and generated the sacrifice, he who alone is God above all gods – who is the God to whom we shall offer sacrifice?

May he not hurt us, he who is the begetter of the earth, or he, the righteous, who begot the heaven; he who also begot the bright and mighty waters – who is the God to whom we shall offer sacrifice?

Prajapati, no other than thou embraces all these created things. May that be ours which we desire when sacrificing to thee; may we be lords of wealth!

(X, 129)

An often-quoted verse declares succinctly: 'Truth is One, though the wise call it by various names' (I, 164, 46).

The above verse has been cited as an example by monistic interpreters of an obvious development in the *Rig Veda* from pantheism to a monistic philosophy. A monistic concept is also present in the following verse: 'Priests and poets with words make into many the hidden reality which is but one' (X, 14).

It is this monistic philosophy that is fully discussed and expounded in the last sections of the four *Vedas*, the *Upanishads*.

The *Vedas* are thought to have been completed, as mentioned, by 600 B.C. In them we possess a vast body of literature that had its beginnings at the dawn of history. Expressed in eloquent poetry and poetic prose, we find hymns of praise to the dawn and to various aspects of Nature; appeals to the various gods; descriptions of sacrificial and sexual rites; magic spells to frighten away ghosts; comments on priests who become drunk on the soma offered in the sacrifices; directions for casting a spell on an adulterer; *mantras* to be uttered during sexual intercourse so that pregnancy might result; *mantras* to be uttered so that pregnancy might not result; actions to be performed if one wished to beget a son with a fair complexion; prayers for rain and for the wealth of many cows. In the *Vedas* we also see the emergence of new gods and the decline of others, and are presented with noble moral ideas about righteousness and purity of life, thoughts on rebirth, and the escaping of rebirth through Yoga practice – from polytheistic to monotheistic and monistic teachings, and lofty metaphysical concepts, almost every thought of man can be found in the Indo-Aryan *Vedas*.

Not so long after the *Vedas* were completed, six systems of philosophy were developed. The six systems of Indian philosophy are usually discussed together since they are interdependent and have their common origin in the *Vedas*. Called the *sad darsanas* – *sad* meaning 'six', and the Sanskrit word *darsana* deriving from the root *dris,* 'to see' – the *sad darsanas* are the six 'insights' or 'points of view'. Complementing each other, and containing cross-references throughout, the six *darsanas* constitute the classical philosophical systems of India. Instead of being regarded as six separate systems, they should be seen as six perspectives on the same doctrine. The Indian holds that the six systems recognize the paramount authority of the *Vedas*. The *Vedas* are the tree, the *darsanas* the branches.

The six systems have identical aims. They all point the way toward union with the Universal Soul, and reveal how the shackles that bind man can be broken through *jnana* (knowledge).

The 'points of view' proceed in closely linked pairs: *Nyaya* and *Vaisheshika, Samkhya* and *Yoga, Purvamimamsa* and *Vedanta.*

The *Nyaya* system was founded by Gautama, who is thought to have lived in the third century B.C. It deals mainly with logic, employing a syllogistic form of argument much like the syllogism of the Greek philosopher Aristotle, except that Gautama's argument consists of five propositions rather than three.

The *Vaisheshika* was founded by Kanada, who is also thought to have lived in the third century B.C. It expounds an atomic theory of the universe, in which it is held that the material world is built up of countless and infinitely small atoms.

The *Samkhya* system was founded by Kapila, who is thought to have lived in the sixth or perhaps even the seventh century B.C. The *Samkhya* is accepted as the oldest of the six 'points of view', and is the most elaborate. Of special interest is its theory of the three *gunas,* or qualities, inherent in *prakriti,* the material substance of the phenomenal universe. In classical Indian literature we often find the three *gunas* mentioned. They are *sattva,* the noble quality of goodness and the higher aspects of mind; *rajas,* the quality of energy and activity; and *tamas,* the quality of darkness and inertia. The three *gunas* are found in man's body as well as in his mind. From *sattva* wisdom and spiritual awakening are produced; from *rajas* comes unrest; from *tamas* come ignorance and delusion.

The *Yoga* system, founded by Patanjali, is a complementary 'point of view' to the *Samkhya* system. The *Yoga* system mentioned here includes all Patanjali's teachings, as preserved for us in his *Yoga Sutras.* One part of these teachings is the system of eight *angas,* or limbs, which Patanjali devised, and which has stood the tests of time and experience. Through the ages, it has been regarded as providing the ideal sequence for applying the different yogic techniques. It is interesting to note that earlier a similar six-step programme was recorded in the *Maitra Upanishad* (VI, 18). This particular system was designed so that the practitioner might attain realization of *Brahman,* the Infinity of Vedantic philosophy. Patanjali's eight-step system can also be adopted for this purpose, as has been done by many past and present-day teachers. By following the actual rules set out in the *Yoga Sutras,* one may come to a direct experience of the Self, leaving all abstract philosophical problems behind.

In compiling his *Yoga Sutras,* Patanjali has drawn upon the great body of sacred Indian writings. The philosophical framework in which his teachings are set is, in broad outline, *Samkhya* philosophy, with the important difference that Patanjali's is obviously theistic. Those of his *sutras* that deal with the *siddhis,* or supernatural powers, said to be developed by the advanced *Yoga* student, have been especially controversial. Even though Patanjali warns (*Yoga Sutras,* III, 38) that these powers are obstacles to ultimate success in Yoga, credulous persons have searched – in vain – for *gurus* (teachers) who could help them attain these *siddhis.* Enlightened persons, however, will not take these *sutras* in their literal sense, but rather as metaphors.

The *Purvamimamsa* 'point of view' was founded by Jaimini, who is thought to have lived about 400 B.C. The *Purvamimamsa* stresses the importance of the Vedic rituals and their precise execution. It penetrates into the meaning of *dharma* (righteousness).

Vedanta was founded by Badarayana, who is thought to have lived about 200 B.C. Badarayana is the author of the *Brahma Sutra,* a summary of the teachings of the *Upanishads. Vedanta* is based on the *Upanishads,* the *Bhagavad Gita,* and the *Brahma Sutra.* As the *Bhagavad Gita* and the *Brahma Sutra* are based on the *Upanishads, Vedanta* proclaims, in essence, the philosophy of the *Upanishads.* This is also indicated by the name of the system, as the word *Vedanta* means 'end of the *Vedas',* and the *Upanishads* are the end, or conclusion, of the *Vedas.*

Of the six systems, *Vedanta* has been, and still is, the most influential philosophical 'point of view'. It has attracted many brilliant minds, of which the greatest undoubtedly was Sankaracharya (A.D. 788-820), who can be called the second father of the *Vedanta* system. His name has become synonymous with *Vedanta.* Sankaracharya's exalted expositions, proclaiming Oneness, will be further dealt with in the next chapter.

The religion based on the *Vedas,* as well as on many supporting classical works – among which the beautiful *Bhagavad Gita* takes a special place – is Hinduism. It is, in all its forms, by far the most significant religion in India today. Hindus believe that the *Vedas* were revealed through divine inspiration.

The highest teaching of the *Vedas,* or more precisely, of the *Upanishads,* is that all is *Brahman,* Universal Spirit. This Upanishadic doctrine teaches that the whole world, and all that is in it, is but a manifestation of the all-pervading *Brahman.* Everything in Hinduism can be reduced to this basic monistic thought. The ultimate goal of the study and practice of Hinduism is to come to this knowledge, which once gained, results in *moksha* (freedom).

In Hinduism the formless *Brahman* is given form as different gods. Evolved from the original deities of the *Vedas,* three major gods now make up the trinity of Hinduism. The impersonal is made personal in Brahma, the god of creation, Vishnu, the god of preservation, and Shiva, the god of destruction, or transformation.

CHAPTER TEN

The Upanishads

The *Upanishads* form the foundation of all yogic teachings. Although there are in existence over two hundred *Upanishads,* not all of them are regarded as authentic. Indian tradition holds that the original *Upanishads* number one hundred and eight. These are all listed in the *Muktika Upanishad,* which states that study of all one hundred and eight will lead to freedom.

The word *upanishad* literally means 'to sit down near'; the student sat at the feet of the master and from his mouth learned the ageless wisdom. The authorship of the *Upanishads* is anonymous. Its subject matter is *Brahman* – the Ultimate Reality underlying all manifestations of life – and the central message of these cherished philosophical treatises is that the individual self is identical with the Universal Self, or *Brahman.*

Of the great number of authentic *Upanishads* – all thought to have been composed before the sixth century B.C. ten or eleven are regarded as the principal ones. The philosophy taught in the *Upanishads* seems, on first acquaintance, not to be entirely consistent. The varying accounts of the creation of the world, for instance, are examples of inconsistency. Various strands of philosophical thought stand side by side, but this perhaps could not be otherwise, since the *Upanishads* form part of the *Vedas,* the sacred scriptures that vary so widely in character. A sympathetic interpretation is required.

Throughout the ages, learned commentators have provided such interpretations. Of these, Sankaracharya, who was born in 788 A.D. in Kaladi, has been by far the most influential. A sage of great mystical insight, Sankaracharya found in the *Upanishads* a consistent philosophy of nondualistic thought. He wrote brilliant commentaries on the eleven major *Upanishads*, in which he shows that the fundamental teaching of the scriptures is that all is *Brahman*. In his work, *Viveka Chudamani*, or 'The Crest Jewel of Wisdom', he states (229): 'It is through ignorance only that this universe appears as having many forms, but when all erroneous ideas have been rejected, all this will be seen as *Brahman*.'

Such a monistic thought is indeed to be found in the *Upanishads*, for example: '*Brahman* is everywhere, upon the right, upon the left, above, below, behind, and in front. The world is but *Brahman*' (*Mundaka Upanishad*, II, ii, 11).

The individual self is identical with *Brahman*: 'The knowledge that *Brahman* and *atman* [the self] are one and the same is true knowledge, and according to the Vedic teachings' (*Viveka Chudamani*, 204).

'In the beginning, son, there was only Being, one without a second', spoke Uddalaka to his son Svetaketu in the *Chandogya Upanishad*. 'Some say there was only nonbeing, and that from nonbeing, Being was born' (VI, ii, 1). 'But how could that be true, son? How could that which is, spring from that which is not? No, son, in the beginning there was Being only, one without a second' (VI, ii, 2). Here we have an important theme of the *Upanishads* – that something cannot arise from nothing. The universe and all that it contains is not a mere accident, but is an emanation of *Brahman*, the Causeless Cause. The law of cause and effect is a manifestation of *Brahman*, but *Brahman* transcends causality. The intellect cannot form a clear conception of something causeless, but then *Brahman* is beyond the grasp of the intellect. *Brahman* is, always was, and always will be. In this world of ceaseless change, the endless number of forms and modes of expression are all manifestations of *Brahman*. A spiritual unity underlies the physical diversity of the world.

Various words – such as Self, That, and Spirit – are frequently used to indicate *Brahman*, but ultimately *Brahman* is indescribable. *Brahman* is beyond all limiting qualifications. As *Brahman* is everything, there is nothing with which it can be compared. No description of *Brahman* can ever be adequate. If one attempted to define *Brahman*, asserting '*Brahman* is this,' or '*Brahman* is this,' the definition would have to be refuted as being either incorrect or incomplete. Hence the famous negative description of *Brahman* in the *Brihadaranyaka Upanishad*: '*neti, neti* (not this, not this).'

In reality, *Brahman* is all that exists, and all that exists is *Brahman*. *Brahman* is omnipresent Being manifesting Itself eternally: 'The Self is one, supreme, the Self of all beings. Though one, It takes the shape of the many. The wise who discover It within, rejoice; who else can rejoice?' (*Katha Upanishad*, II, ii, 12).

The *Upanishads* exclaim: '*Tat tvam asi* – (That thou art!)' To come to this realization is the aim of the Jnana Yoga student.

KATHA UPANISHAD

Vajasravasa, desiring heaven, performed the sacrifice of giving away all his property.   (I, i, 1)

His son Nachiketa, though still a boy, thought to himself: 'Surely, this which he is earning cannot be much of a heaven – his cows can no longer eat, nor can they drink, nor give milk, nor calve.'
(I, i, 2–3)

Going to his father, he asked: 'To whom will you give me, Father?' When he had asked three times, his father told him angrily: 'I shall give you to Death!'   (I, i, 4)

Nachiketa thought: 'Men are mortal. Whether I die now or later is ultimately of little concern. What would happen if Death gets me now?'   (I, i, 5)

Not wanting his regretful father to go back on his word, he said: 'Think of those who went before us, as well as of those who are with us now. A corn ripens, is cut, and is born again.'   (I, i, 6)

Nachiketa went into the forest, and entered the house of Yama, the King of Death, where he fasted as he waited.   (I, i, 7)

Yama appeared, and spoke to Nachiketa: 'I bow to you, O holy man! Three days you have lived in my house without eating or drinking. For my sake, please choose three boons.'   (I, i, 9)

Nachiketa said: 'O Yama, as my first boon I choose a reconciliation with my father; may he be cheerful, and bear me no grudge when we meet again.'   (I, i, 10)

Yama said: 'Your wish is granted. He will recognize you and be friendly towards you. On realizing that you are free from the jaws of death, he will again sleep peacefully at night, and he will be reconciled with you.'   (I, i, 11)

Nachiketa said: 'Because you are absent, there is no fear in the kingdom of heaven. All rejoice in heaven, being beyond hunger, thirst, and sorrow.'   (I, i, 12)

'O Death! You know the sacrifice of Fire which leads to heaven. Explain to me the secret of that Fire, for I am full of faith. That secret I choose as my second boon.'   (I, i, 13)

Yama said: 'Listen! I shall explain it to you. It is locked within the hearts of the wise.'   (I, i, 14)

'The Fire feeds on study, meditation, and practice. He who performs this triple duty, and knows the Fire to be born of *Brahman,* attains everlasting peace.'   (I, i, 17)

'He who performs the three duties throws off, though still on earth, the chains of death. Overcoming sorrow, he enjoys heaven.'

(I, i, 18)

'Knowledge of this Fire, which leads to heaven, is your second boon. I shall name it after you, Nachiketa. Now choose the third boon.'   (I, i, 19)

Nachiketa said: 'There is controversy about man's condition after he dies. Some say he continues to exist, others say he does not. Explain this to me as my third boon.'   (I, i, 20)

Yama said: 'On this question even the gods had doubts. It is difficult to understand. Choose something else, Nachiketa. Please do not force me to explain.'   (I, i, 21)

Nachiketa said: 'O Death! You state that even the gods had doubts, that it is a question difficult to understand. But who can explain it better than you? What other boon is as great?' (I, i, 22)

Yama said: 'Take long-living sons and grandsons, herds of cattle, horses, and elephants, gold. Take a kingdom; live on earth as long as you wish.'   (I, i, 23)

'Choose anything you want, O Nachiketa! The greatest kingdom, a long life, anything you desire.'   (I, i, 24)

'Whatever pleasure there is, fine maidens with chariots and musical instruments, delights beyond dreams. They will be yours, but do not ask me about life after death.'   (I, i, 25)

Nachiketa said: 'O Death! These things are temporary. They exhaust the senses. Even the longest life passes. Keep those horses, keep for yourself all those dances and songs.'   (I, i, 26)

'Wealth does not bring happiness. Since I have found favour with you, I shall get wealth and long life. However, I shall not change the boon that I have asked.'   (I, i, 27)

'What mortal man, seeing immortality, having the chance of immortality, would prefer a mere long life, albeit filled with sexual and other delights?'   (I, i, 28)

'O Death! Tell me of this eternity about which there is so much doubt. This is the boon I insist upon.'   (I, i, 29)

Yama said: 'The good is one thing, the pleasant another. Both bind man. He who strives for the good, attains the Highest; he who strives for the pleasant, falls by the wayside.'   (I, ii, 1)

'Each man faces both. The wise man discriminates, and pursues the good; greed and desires of the flesh drive the ignorant to the pleasant.'   (I, ii, 2)

'O Nachiketa! After examining the temporary pleasures, you have rejected them. You have not turned into the road to wealth, the road in which many become bogged.'   (I, ii, 3)

'Wide apart these roads are; one is named ignorance, the other wisdom. Not deceived by the promise of wealth you decided on wisdom, O Nachiketa!'   (I, ii, 4)

'Fools live in darkness. Staggering to and fro, they boast of their supposed wisdom, blind leading blind.'   (I, ii, 5)

'What does he who is entangled in greed know about eternity? "This is the only world that exists!" he cries, and because of this I mow him down again and again.'   (I, ii, 6)

'Many have never heard of the Self; many, having heard, do not comprehend. Rare is the expounder, and rare the hearer; rare is he who knows the Self through instruction from a teacher.'
                    (I, ii, 7)

'Knowledge of the Self, being hard to attain, cannot be taught by one with ordinary mind. But when it is expounded by him who has become one with *Brahman,* there remains no more doubt. The Self is slighter than the slightest, and transcends argument.' (I, ii, 8)

'Knowledge of the Self cannot be arrived at by reasoning alone. It can be found, O beloved, when taught by someone who has this knowledge. You are, indeed, a true seeker. If only inquirers like you were always sent me!' (I, ii, 9)

'The wise man, by concentrating on the Self, realizes that ancient Self, difficult to imagine, more difficult to understand. He will pass beyond joy and sorrow.' (I, ii, 12)

'The wise man, being instructed and comprehending, separates nature from the Self. He lives forever and rejoices forever in *Brahman.*' (I, ii, 13)

Nachiketa said: 'Tell me, O Death! What is other than right and wrong, other than cause and effect, other than past and future?' (I, ii, 14)

Yama said: 'It is *Om,* expounded by the *Vedas,* the purpose of austerities and the goal of purity.' (I, ii, 15)

'*Om* is indeed *Brahman*. It is the highest. He who knows this word can obtain all he desires.' (I, ii, 16)

'*Om* is the foundation. He who finds this foundation is worthy of the company of saints.' (I, ii, 17)

'The all-knowing Self is not born and does not die. It is not caused, and It causes not. Eternal, everlasting and imperishable, It is not killed when the body is killed.' (I, ii, 18)

'The Self, smaller than the smallest, greater than the greatest, lives within the hearts of all. When a man becomes free of desires, and purifies his mind and senses, he will behold the glory of the Self, and go beyond sorrow.' (I, ii, 20)

'Though seated, the Self goes far; though at rest, It moves everywhere. Who but me, King of Death, can understand this effulgent Being which is joy and goes beyond joy?' (I, ii, 21)

'He who knows the Self, formless among the formed, unchanging among the changing, all-pervading and supreme, he transcends all grief.' (I, ii, 22)

'Knowledge of this Self cannot be obtained through study of the scriptures, nor through intellectual investigation, nor through discourse. It comes to the man who ardently longs for it; to him the true nature of the Self is revealed.' (I, ii, 23)

'Know the Self as the rider of the body, the chariot; intellect is the charioteer; mind, the reins.' (I, iii, 3)

'The senses are the horses; desired objects, the roads. The wise call the Self the Enjoyer when It is joined to body, mind and senses.' (I, iii, 4)

'When the intellect, living in a mind which is easily distracted, loses its discrimination, the senses become unmanageable, like the restive horses of the charioteer.' (I, iii, 5)

'But when the intellect, living in a well-controlled mind, possesses sharp discrimination, the senses can be restrained, like the obeying horses of the charioteer.' (I, iii, 6)

'He whose intellect firmly grasps the reins of the mind, reaches the supreme goal of the journey, all-pervading *Brahman*.' (I, iii, 9)

'The Self, hidden in all being, is not seen by all; but It is seen by the sages of concentrated mind and subtle intellect.' (I, iii, 12)

'The wise man merges speech in mind, mind in intellect, intellect in manifested nature, nature in *Brahman*, and thus finds Peace.'
(I, iii, 13)

'Arise! Awake! Learn at the feet of the master. The sages say the path is difficult, sharp as the edge of a razor.' (I, iii, 14)

'He who knows the soundless, formless, intangible, deathless, tasteless, undecaying, odourless, beginningless, endless, unchanging *Brahman*, he escapes the jaws of Death.' (I, iii, 15)

Yama said : 'The Self-Existent made the senses turn outward; accordingly, man looks outward, and sees not what is within. Every so often a man, desiring immortality, looks inward, and beholds the Self.' (II, i, 1)

'The ignorant follow the desires of the flesh, and sink into the swamp of death; but the wise, searching for what is eternal, seek not the things that decay.' (II, i, 2)

'He who knows that the individual self, the enjoyer of the results of action, is the Universal Self, in which rest present, past, and future, he has no fear.' (II, i, 5)

'That Being, which is the inborn power of all powers, which is embodied in the elements, and which is living in the lotus of the heart, that is Self.'   (II, i, 7)

'Only by the purified mind can the indivisible *Brahman* be attained. He who sees only multiplicity in *Brahman* wanders from death to death.'   (II, i, 11)

'As rain falling on the mountain top runs off in all directions, so he who sees only multiplicity runs in all directions.'   (II, i, 14)

'As pure water poured into pure water remains pure, so he remains pure who knows the unity of *Brahman*.'   (II, i, 15)

'He who meditates on pure Consciousness, abiding in the body, the city of eleven gates, grieves no more. He becomes forever free.'
(II, ii, 1)

'The Self is the sun in the sky, the air in space, the fire on the altar, the guest in the house; he is all men and all gods. The Self lives in the water and upon the earth, in truth and in greatness. Omnipresent Reality is the Self.'   (II, ii, 2)

'O Nachiketa! I shall tell you of the eternal Spirit, and of what happens after death.'   (II, ii, 6)

'Some enter, through the womb, into living beings; others enter matter, according to their deeds and knowledge.'   (II, ii, 7)

'As fire, though one, takes the shape of whatever it consumes, so the Self, though one, takes the shape of whatever It enters. It exists also outside.'   (II, ii, 9)

'As the sun, lighting the world, is not affected by the impurities it shines upon, so the Self, dwelling in all things, is not touched by evil, existing outside it.'   (II, ii, 11)

'The Self is one, supreme, the Self of all beings. Though one, It takes the shape of the many. The wise who discover It within, rejoice; who else can rejoice?'   (II, ii, 12)

'Eternal among things transient, though one, It fulfills the desires of the many. The wise who discover It within, find peace : Who else can find peace?'   (II, ii, 13)

'The universe is a tree with its roots above and its branches spread on the ground. The roots spring from *Brahman*, eternal Spirit. In That all things live, and none can go beyond It; That is Self.'
(II, iii, 1)

'The organs of perception have their separate origin; their action and nonaction are distinct from the Self. The wise man, knowing this, grieves no more.'   (II, iii, 6)

'When the sense organs and the mind become still, when the intellect does not waver, then man comes to the highest state.'
(II, iii, 10)

'The constant and firm control of senses and mind is called Yoga. Once he reaches the highest state, the yogi can do no wrong.'
(II, iii, 11)

'*Brahman* cannot be known through discourse, nor reached by the mind, nor seen by the eyes. It can only be taught through the experience of those who affirm Its existence.'   (II, iii, 12)

'First, the existence of the individual self must be realized; this then leads to knowledge of its true nature, which is pure Existence.'
(II, iii, 13)

'The mortal, who has killed all desires, though still in the body, attains *Brahman*; finite becomes infinite.'   II, iii, 14)

'When the ties of ignorance which bind the heart are cut, then mortal becomes immortal. This is the highest teaching of the scriptures.'   (II, iii, 15)

Nachiketa, having received from the King of Death this knowledge, and the whole process of Yoga, became free from evil and death, and attained *Brahman*; he who does likewise, finds the innermost Self.   (II, iii, 18)

ISA UPANISHAD

The Self, though unmoving, moves faster than the mind. The senses cannot reach It, for the Self runs before them. Unmoving, I overtakes others who are running. Out of Self come all activities. (4

Unmoving, It moves; It is far away, yet near; It is inside all this and outside all this.   (5

The wise man who sees all creatures in the Self, and the Self in all creatures, knows no sorrow.   (6

What delusion, what sorrow can there be for the seer who behold the unity of life?   (7

One thing is obtained from knowledge, another from ignorance The wise taught us this.   (10

He who can distinguish between knowledge and ignorance, he overcomes death springing from ignorance, and through knowledge obtains immortal life. (11)

KENA UPANISHAD

The student asked : 'What has set my mind into motion? What directs the *prana* in me? What makes me speak? What god directs my eyes and ears?' (I, 1)

The teacher replied : 'It thinks in all minds, lives in all lives, speaks through all mouths, looks through all eyes, and hears through all ears. The wise detach the Self from the senses and, renouncing the world, attain immortality.' (I, 2)

'The eye cannot see It, and the mind cannot know It. We do not know It, and we cannot teach It. It is different from the known as well as the unknown. Thus we have been told by the ancient teachers.' (I, 3–4)

'Know that as *Brahman* which cannot be expressed by speech, but by which speech is expressed; not that which is worshipped by ignorant people.' (I, 5)

'Know that as *Brahman* which cannot be thought by the mind, but by which the mind thinks; not that which is worshipped by ignorant people.' (I, 6)

'Know that as *Brahman* which cannot be seen by the eye, but by which the eye sees; not that which is worshipped by ignorant people.' (I, 7)

'Know that as *Brahman* which cannot be heard by the ear, but by which the ear hears; not that which is worshipped by ignorant people.' (I, 8)

'Know that as *Brahman* without which life cannot live, that which makes everything alive; not that which is worshipped by ignorant people.' (I, 9)

The teacher said : 'If you think you know much about *Brahman*, then surely you know little; you only know It through a mind conditioned by man and circumstance.' (II, 1)

In ancient times the gods of nature became convinced they were almighty. (III, 1)

Spirit, understanding the mistaken notion of the gods, appeared.
The gods did not know who Spirit was.   (III, 2)

They said to Agni, the god of fire: 'Agni, find out who this
mysterious Spirit is!'   (III, 3)

Agni ran to Spirit and stated: 'I am Agni.'   (III, 4)

Spirit asked: 'What can you do?'
Agni said: 'I can burn anything and everything in this world.'
                                                              (III, 5)

Spirit put down a straw, and spoke to Agni: 'Burn this.'
Agni engulfed the piece of straw, but could not burn it. Thereupon
he hastened back to the gods and confessed: 'I cannot find out
who this mysterious Spirit is.'   (III, 6)

The gods then said to Vaya, the god of air: 'Vaya, find out who
this mysterious spirit is!'   (III, 7)

Vaya ran to Spirit and stated: 'I am Vaya.'   (III, 8)

Spirit asked: 'What can you do?'
Vaya said: 'I can blow away anything and everything in this
world.'   (III, 9)

Spirit put down a straw, and spoke to Vaya: 'Blow this away.'
With all his might, Vaya threw himself upon the piece of straw
but he could not move it. Thereupon he hastened back to the
gods, and confessed: 'I cannot find out who this mysterious
Spirit is.'   (III, 10)

Then the gods said to Indra, the great god of light: 'Indra, find
out who this mysterious Spirit is.' Indra ran to Spirit but Spirit
disappeared instantly.   (III, 11)

Indra saw in the sky Uma, the beautiful goddess of wisdom,
daughter of the Himalayas. Indra went to her, and asked: 'Who
is this mysterious Spirit?'   (III, 12)

Uma replied: 'That Spirit is *Brahman*; through the greatness of
Brahman alone can you attain greatness.' Indra then understood
that Spirit was *Brahman*.   (IV, 1)

Now listen to the instruction concerning *Brahman* for the individual self. The power of the mind belongs to *Brahman*. The
seeker attains *Brahman* through the mind. He should meditate on
Brahman with all aspects of his mind.   (IV, 5)

This knowledge is founded on austerity, self-control, and meditation. It is supported by the *Vedas,* and Truth is its abode.   (IV, 8)

He who knows this *Upanishad* overcomes all evil, and forever
exists in the infinite *Brahman.*   (IV, 9)

PRASNA UPANISHAD

Students, bringing offerings and faith, approached the sage Pip-
palada and asked him for instruction in the knowledge of the
supreme *Brahman.*   (I, 1)

The sage said : 'Stay with me for one year, practising austerity,
continence, and 'faith; then you may ask what questions you like.
If I can, I shall answer you.'   (I, 2)

When the year was up, one student asked : 'Sir, how did all these
creatures come into being?'   (I, 3)

The sage said : 'The Creator, having performed austerities, in
meditation created a couple—*prana,* the manly life-force, and
rayi, the female food. He willed that this couple should produce
many creatures.'   (I, 4)

'*Prana,* the life-force, is the sun; *rayi,* food, is the moon. Everything that has form is food.'   (I, 5)

'The rising sun shines on all beings in the east, and fills them with
energy. Then it illuminates the other regions, engulfing all beings
with its life-giving rays.'   (I, 6)

Another student asked : 'Sir, how many different powers hold this
body together? How many manifest their power through it? Of
these, which is paramount?'   (II, 1)

The sage said : 'The powers are ether, air, fire, water, and earth.
These five elements form the physical body. Also present are
speech, mind, eye, and ear. All these powers proclaimed they
upheld the body.'   (II, 2)

'*Prana,* the primal energy, told them : "Do not deceive yourselves.
It is I alone, dividing myself into five streams, who support the
body and keep it together." But the powers were sceptical.' (II, 3)

'*Prana,* in justification, rose as if about to leave the body. But as
prana rose, the others had to rise too. When *prana* settled down
again, the others could settle down. As bees follow their queen

when she goes out, and return when she returns, so it is with speech, mind, eye and ear. Convinced, they began to praise *prana.*'
(II, 4)

'*Prana* burns in the fire, shines in the sun, is in the rain, the greatest of gods, the air, the earth, the food. It is that which has shape, and that which has no shape. It is immortality.' (II, 5)

'As spokes in the hub of the wheel, all is fixed in *prana*—the *Vedas,* the sacrifices, the warriors, the priests.' (II, 6)

Then another student asked : 'Sir, from where was this *prana* born? How does it enter the body? How does it live in the body after it has divided itself? How does it depart? How does it support what is outside and what is inside?' (III, 1)

The sage replied : 'You ask very difficult questions; you must be a sincere seeker. Therefore I shall answer you.' (III, 2)

'*Prana* is born of *Brahman.* As shadow falls from man, so *prana* falls from *Brahman. Prana* enters the body to fulfill the desires of the mind.' (III, 3)

'As a king employs officials to govern over parts of his kingdom, so *prana* employs secondary *pranas,* each having its own function.'
(III, 4)

'*Prana* itself moves through the mouth and nose, and lives in the eye and the ear. It engages *apana* in the organs of excretion and procreation. In the middle of the body *samana* reigns, directing digestion and assimilation.' (III, 5)

'The Self lives in the lotus of the heart, from where spring one hundred and one channels, each of these channels branching into one hundred channels, and these again into seventy-two thousand smaller channels. In all these channels, *vyana* rules.' (III, 6)

'Ascending through one of these, *udana,* at the moment of death, conducts the virtuous man to his reward, and the sinful man to his punishment; those who were both virtuous and sinful are brought back to the world of men.' (III, 7)

'The sun is the *prana* of the external world; it rises, activating the *prana* in the eye of man. Earth controls *apana*; ether between heaven and earth maintains *samana*; the wind, *vyana.*' (III, 8)

'*Udana* takes up the mind's desire at the moment of death, returns to *prana,* and *prana,* guided by *udana,* leads the soul to the world it has earned.' (III, 10)

'He who knows the source of *prana,* its entry into the body, how it dwells after its fivefold division, its internal and external relation, he obtains immortality; verily, he obtains immortality.'   (III, 12)

Another student said : 'Sir, once a prince asked me whether I knew the Person with sixteen parts. I did not know, and I could not tell him a lie. Verily he who tells lies perishes, root and all. Tell me, please, where does this Person dwell?'   (VI, 1)

The sage said : 'The Person with the sixteen parts lives in this body.'   (VI, 2)

'That Person reflected : "By the departure of which shall I depart, and the staying of which shall I stay?" '   (VI, 3)

'He then created *prana*; from *prana,* desire; from desire, ether; from ether, air; from air, fire; from fire, water; from water, earth; from earth, senses; from senses, mind; from mind, food; from food, virility; from virility, austerity; from austerity, the *Vedas*; from the *Vedas,* sacrifice; from sacrifice, world; from world, names.' (VI, 4)

'As rivers flow into the sea, losing their names and forms, they are called only the sea; so these sixteen parts, created by that Person, flow into that Person, and they are called the Self. Then the seer becomes free of parts, and immortal. This is my teaching :   (VI, 5)

'Know the Self, which is the goal of knowledge, and in which the parts rest firmly, as the spokes in the hub of the wheel. Know the Self, and die no more.'   (VI, 6)

'I have told you all that can be said about the Self, the supreme *Brahman*; beyond this there is naught.'   (VI, 7)

The students worshipped the sage and said : 'You are indeed our father. You have led us across the sea of ignorance.
                'We bow to the great *rishis* !
                'We bow to the great *rishis* !'   (VI, 8)

MUNDAKA UPANISHAD

The first of the gods was Brahma, maker and protector of the universe. He revealed the Knowledge of *Brahman,* the foundation of all knowledge, to his eldest son Atharva.   (I, i, 1)

In times long ago, Atharva told it to Angir, who passed it on to Satyavaka, member of the Bharadvaya family. Satyavaka taught it to Angiras.   (I, i, 2)

Saunaka, the famous householder, approached Angiras and asked respectfully: 'Holy Sir, what is that which, when known, makes us know everything?' (I, i, 3)

Angiras replied: 'The knowers of *Brahman* tell us that there are two kinds of knowledge – the higher knowledge and the lower knowledge.' (I, i, 4)

'The lower is the knowledge of the *Rig-*, the *Yajur-*, the *Sama-*, and the *Atharva-Veda*, of phonetics, ceremonials, grammar, etymology, meter and astronomy; the higher is the knowledge by which one attains the everlasting *Brahman*.' (I, i, 5)

'Through the higher knowledge the wise behold that which can neither be seen nor grasped, that which has neither eyes nor ears, hands nor feet, which is uncaused, all-prevalent, omnipresent yet immeasurably minute, imperishable, and the source of all beings.'
(I, i, 6)

'As the web springs from the spider and is withdrawn again, as the plant springs from the earth, as hairs from man's body, so the world springs from *Brahman*.' (I, i, 7)

'*Brahman's* reflection made *prakriti* [primal matter] ready for manifestation; from *prakriti* came *prana*; from *prana*, mind; from mind, the elements; from the elements, the worlds; from the worlds, *karma* [actions]; from *karma*, their immortal results.' (I, i, 8)

'*Brahman* knows all and understands all; *Brahman* is knowledge itself. From *Brahman* spring Brahma, name, form, and food.'
(I, i, 9)

'*Brahman* lives in the heart. It is the support and centre of everything that moves and breathes. That which is both the gross and the subtle, which is supreme and beyond learning, know that to be your Self.' (II, ii, 1)

'Take the *Upanishads*, the great weapon, as the bow; lay against it the arrow of devotion. Pulling the sharp arrow back with a mind concentrated on *Brahman*, hit the target – the Imperishable.'
(II, ii, 3)

'*Om* is the bow; *atman*, the individual self, is the arrow; *Brahman*, the Universal Self, is the target. Aim with undistracted mind, and become one with *Brahman*, just as the arrow merges with the target.' (II, ii, 4)

'In *Brahman* are woven heaven, earth, and space, mind and senses. Know the Self, and discard all else. *Brahman* is the bridge to immortality.' (II, ii, 5)

'As the spokes of the wheel meet in the hub, so the many forms of *Brahman* centre in the lotus of the heart where the channels meet. Meditate on the Self as *Om,* and cross the sea of darkness.'
(II, ii, 6)

'Neither sun, moon, stars, fire, nor lightning light *Brahman.* When *Brahman* shines, everything shines; everything in the world reflects *Brahman's* light.' (II, ii, 10)

'*Brahman* is everywhere, upon the right, upon the left, above, below, behind, and in front. The world is but *Brahman.*' (II, ii, 11)

'This Self, residing within the lotus of the heart, is found by the ascetics through consistency, truthfulness, intelligence, and continence.' (III, i, 5)

'Truth alone triumphs, not falsehood. The path to bliss is paved with truth. Along it, the seers, with desires mastered, travel to the abode of Truth.' (III, i, 6)

'The eyes cannot see *Brahman,* nor can tongue speak It, nor the senses reach It. *Brahman* cannot be discovered by penance or sacrificial ritual. When the heart has become pure, and the mind grown still, then formless Truth is revealed.' (III, i, 8)

'The Self shines in this body where the *prana* divides into the five streams. Pervading mind and senses, the Self shines for the pure intellect.' (III, i, 9)

'The sage knows That which contains the universe. The man who, having overcome desires, worships the sage, will escape from births and deaths.' (III, ii, 1)

'The Self cannot be known by the weak, nor by the half-hearted, nor through austerity without aim. But the wise man who is strong, earnest, and sincere, he will enter the abode of *Brahman.*'
(III, ii, 4)

'Having attained the Self, the seers are satisfied with their Knowledge. Free from passion, tranquil, they behold the omnipresent Self on all sides. Those wise men, with concentrated minds, enter the All.' (III, ii, 5)

'Verily, he who knows the supreme *Brahman*, becomes *Brahman*. No one is born in his family ignorant of *Brahman*. He goes beyond sorrow, beyond sin. Liberated from the entanglements of the heart, he becomes immortal.'   (III, ii, 9)

AITAREYA UPANISHAD

In the beginning this was the Self, one only. Nothing else moved. He thought : 'Let me create the worlds.'   (I, i, 1)

He created these worlds : the world of clouds, the world of light rays, the world of earth, and the world of waters. The clouds are above heaven, and supported by heaven. The light rays are space. On the earth are mortals. Beneath are the waters.   (I, i, 2)

He thought : 'Here are the worlds. Now let me create their rulers.' From the waters, he drew forth the Person and gave Him a form.
(I, i, 3)

He brooded over Him. In the Person a mouth appeared; from the mouth came speech, from speech, fire. A nose formed; from the nostrils came breath, from breath, air. The eyes took shape; from the eyes came sight, from sight, the sun. The ears appeared; from the ears came hearing, from hearing, the quarters of space. The skin grew; from the skin came the hairs, from hairs, plants and trees. The heart formed; from the heart came the mind, from the mind, the moon. The navel appeared; from the navel came the downward breath, *apana*, from *apana*, death. The sex organ formed; from the sex organ came seed, from seed, water.   (I, i, 4)

These gods thus created fell into the great waters. The Self subjected the gods to hunger and thirst. The gods said : 'Find us a place where we may live and eat.'   (I, ii, 1)

The Creator brought them a cow. They said : 'This is not enough for us.' Then He brought them a horse. They said : 'This is not enough for us.'   (I, ii, 2)

Then He brought them a man. The gods said : 'This is well done indeed.' Therefore a man is something well done. He spoke to the gods : 'Enter into your abodes.'   (I, ii, 3)

The god of fire, becoming speech, entered the mouth. Air, becoming breath, entered the nostrils. The sun, becoming sight, entered the eyes. The quarters of space, becoming hearing, entered the ears. Plants and trees, becoming hairs, entered the skin. The moon, becoming mind, entered the heart. Death, becoming *apana,* entered the navel. Water, becoming seed, entered the sex organ.   (I, ii, 4)

Hunger and thirst said : 'For us also find an abode.' The Creator spoke to them : 'I give you a place in all these gods, and you will share with them. Therefore to whatever god an offering is made, hunger and thirst will partake.'   (I, ii, 5)

He thought : 'Here are the worlds, and the rulers of the worlds. I shall create food for them.'   (I, iii, 1)

He brooded over the waters, and from the waters emerged a form. That form was indeed food.   (I, iii, 2)

The food thus created fled from man. Man sought to seize it with speech. But he was not able to seize it with speech. If he had been able to seize it with speech, to talk about it would have been sufficient.   (I, iii, 3)

Man sought to grasp it with breath. But he was not able to grasp it with breath. If he had been able to grasp it with breath, to inhale it would have been sufficient.   (I, iii, 4)

Man sought to grasp it with sight. But he was not able to grasp it with sight. If he had been able to grasp it with sight, to look at it would have been sufficient.   (I, iii, 5)

Man sought to seize it with hearing. But he was not able to seize it with hearing. If he had been able to seize it with hearing, to hear it would have been sufficient.   (I, iii, 6)

Man sought to take hold of it with the skin. But he was not able to take hold of it with the skin. If he had been able to take hold of it with the skin, to touch it would have been sufficient.   (I, iii, 7)

Man sought to grasp it with the mind. But he was not able to grasp it with the mind. If he had been able to grasp it with the mind, to think about it would have been sufficient.   (I, iii, 8)

Man sought to seize it with the sex organ. But he was not able to seize it with the sex organ. If he had been able to seize it with the sex organ, emitting seed would have been sufficient.   (I, iii, 9)

Man then sought to seize it with the downward air, *apana,* and he succeeded. The seizer of food is what this air is. This air is what lives on food.   (I, iii, 10)

The Creator thought : 'How can they exist without Me? Which way shall I enter the body?' He thought : 'If the tongue speaks, the nose smells, the eyes see, the ears hear, the skin feels, the mind thinks, *apana* digests, and the sex organ emits, then how will man know Me?'   (I, iii, 11)

He opened the top of the head, and entered through the opening, which is called the gate of bliss. The Self has three abodes: the conditions of waking, dreaming, and deep sleep.   (I, iii, 12)

Thus manifested as the individual self, He perceived the created beings. What else would one have to say? He saw nothing but all-pervading *Brahman*, and spoke: 'I know *Brahman*.'   (I, iii, 13)

First the self is the seed of man. This seed is the vigour gathered from all the limbs. Man bears the seed in himself. When he ejects his seed into a woman, he gives it a birth. That is the first birth of the self.   (II, i, 1)

The seed becomes part of the woman; because it becomes part of her, it does her no harm. She nourishes this self which has entered her.   (II, i, 2)

Nourish the woman, because she nourishes the seed. After the birth, the father nourishes the child. Nourishing the child, he nourishes himself. That is the second birth of the self.   (II, i, 3)

The son is made the father's substitute for the performing of virtuous acts. When the father has accomplished his duties and exhausted his years, he departs and is born again. That is the third birth of the self.   (II, i, 4)

The sage Vamadeva said: 'While lying in the womb, I knew all the births of the gods. I was confined by a hundred iron prisons, yet I broke free swiftly, like a hawk.'   (II, i, 5)

Thus the sage Vamadeva, endowed with knowledge, became one with *Brahman*. Ascending into the heavenly worlds, he obtained all his desires, and became immortal; yes, became immortal.
    (II, i, 6)

Which is the Self we should meditate upon? Is it He by whom we see, hear, smell, speak, and distinguish the sweet and the bitter?
    (III, i, 1)

He is in the heart and the mind as consciousness, perception, knowledge, wisdom, steadfastness, thought, thoughtfulness, impulse, memory, conception, purpose, life, desire, longing – all these are names of Consciousness.   (III, i, 2)

He is Brahma; He is Indra; He is Prajapati; He is all these gods. He is these five great elements – earth, air, ether, water, light. He is the small and the large creatures, those born of egg, womb, sweat, and soil, horses, cows, men, elephants, whatever breathes, whether moving, or flying, or unmoving. All this is guided by Consciousness, is established in Consciousness. All this is based on Consciousness. *Brahman* is Consciousness.   (III, i, 3)

The sage Vamadeva, knowing Consciousness, soared upward from this world. Obtaining all his desires in the heavenly world, he became immortal; yes, became immortal.   (III, i, 4)

CHANDOGYA UPANISHAD

Om. Once there lived Svetaketu, grandson of Aruna. His father, named Uddalaka, said to him : 'Svetaketu, lead the life of a *brahmacharin* [religious student]; none of our family, son, is a *brahmin* [member of the priestly caste] by birth only.'   (VI, i, 1)

Svetaketu found a teacher and became a student at the age of twelve. He studied the *Vedas*. When he was twenty-four he returned home – conceited, considering himself well-read, and arrogant.

Uddalaka said to him : 'Svetaketu, since you now think that you know so much, did you ever ask for that instruction,   (VI, i, 2)

'by which one hears what cannot be heard, perceives what cannot be perceived, knows what cannot be known?'

Svetaketu asked : 'What is that instruction, Sir?'   (VI, i, 3)

Uddalaka replied : 'Son, as by knowing one clod of clay all things made of clay are known, the difference being only names arising from speech, the truth being that they are clay;   (VI, i, 4)

'as by knowing one nugget of gold all things made of gold are known, the difference being only names arising from speech, the truth being that they are gold;   (VI, i, 5)

'as by knowing one piece of metal all things made of metal are known, the difference being only names arising from speech, the truth being that they are metal – thus, son, is that instruction.'
                    (VI, i, 6)

Svetaketu said : 'Apparently my revered teacher did not know it. For had he known it, surely he would have taught me. Therefore, Sir, please give me that instruction.'
'I shall, son,' Uddalaka said.   (VI, i, 7)

'In the beginning, son, there was only Being, one without a second. Some say that there was only nonbeing, and that from nonbeing Being was born.' (VI, ii, 1)

'But how could that be true, son?' Uddalaka said. 'How could that which is, spring from that which is not? No, son, in the beginning, there was Being only, one without a second.' (VI, ii, 2)

'It thought: "Let Me be many, let Me grow forth." It produced fire. That fire thought: "Let me be many, let me grow forth." It produced water. Therefore, whenever a person is hot and perspires, water is produced on him from the heat of the fire.' (VI, ii, 3)

'Water thought: "Let me be many, let me grow forth." It produced food. Therefore, whenever it rains, food is produced in abundance. So edible food is produced from water alone.'
(VI, ii, 4)

'That Being thought: "Let Me enter these three gods by means of the self, and develop names and forms." ' (VI, iii, 2)

' "Let Me make each of these gods threefold," that Being thought as It entered these gods, and developed names and forms.'
(VI, iii, 3)

'Food when eaten becomes threefold – its greatest portion becomes faeces, its middle portion flesh, its subtlest portion mind.' (VI, v, 1)

'Water when drunk becomes threefold – its grossest portion becomes urine, its middle portion blood, its subtlest portion *prana*.'
(VI, v, 2)

'Fire when absorbed [in heat-generating food] becomes threefold – its grossest portion becomes bones, its middle portion marrow, its subtlest portion speech.' (VI, v, 3)

'Therefore, son, mind comes from food, *prana* from water, and speech from fire.'
'Please, Sir, instruct me further,' said Svetaketu.
'I shall, son,' Uddalaka replied. (VI, v,)

Uddalaka, son of Aruna, spoke to Svetaketu: 'Learn from me the true nature of sleep. When a man here sleeps, then, son, he becomes united with that Being; he has gone to his own Self. Therefore they say that he sleeps, for he has gone to his own.'
(VI, viii,)

'As the tethered bird first flies in every direction and, finding no rest anywhere, finally settles down on the very place where it is fastened, so the mind, son, after flying in every direction, and finding no rest anywhere, finally settles down on *prana*; for indeed, son, mind is fastened to *prana*.   (VI, viii, 2)

'In that which is the subtle essence, in that all that exists has its self. That is Truth. That is Self. That thou art!'
'Please, Sir, instruct me further,' said Svetaketu.
'I shall, son,' Uddalaka replied.   (VI, viii, 7)

'As bees, son, produce honey by gathering the juices from different flowers, and reduce them to one mixture,   (VI, ix, 1)

'and as these juices in the honey have no discrimination, so that they can say: "I am the juice of this or that flower," so indeed, son, all these creatures, though merged in that Being, know not that they are merged in that Being.'   (VI, ix, 2)

'Whatever these creatures are in this world – be it tiger, lion, wolf, boar, worm, fly, gnat or mosquito – that they become again.'
                                                    (VI, ix, 3)

'In that which is the subtle essence, in that all that exists has its self. That is Truth. That is Self. That thou art!'
Please, Sir, instruct me further,' said Svetaketu.
I shall, son,' Uddalaka replied.   (VI, ix, 4)

'These rivers, son, flow – the eastern to the east, the western to the west. They arise from the sea [vapour, clouds, rain] and flow into the sea. They become the sea. As these rivers, while in the sea, do not know "I am this or that river,"   (VI, x, 1)

in the same manner, son, all these creatures, springing from that Being, know not that they have come from the Being. Whatever these creatures are here in this world – be it tiger, lion, wolf, boar, worm, fly, gnat, or mosquito – that they become again.' (VI, x, 2)

In that which is the subtle essence, in that all that exists has its self. That is Truth, That is Self. That thou art!'
Please, Sir, instruct me further,' said Svetaketu.
I shall, son,' Uddalaka replied.   (VI, x, 3)

If you strike at the root of that large tree there, it will lose sap, but it will still live. If you strike at its trunk, it will lose sap, but it will still live. If you strike at its crown, it will lose sap, but it continues to live. The tree is pervaded by the Self, and it stands firm, happily drinking its nourishment.'   (VI, xi, 1)

E

'But if life leaves one of the tree's branches, then that branch withers; if it leaves a second, the second branch withers; if it leaves a third, the third branch withers. If it leaves the whole tree, the whole tree withers. In exactly the same manner, son,' Uddalaka said, 'know this :   (VI, xi, 2)

'Verily, this body withers and dies when deprived of the Self, but the Self does not die. In that which is the subtle essence, in that all that exists has its self. That is Truth. That is Self. That thou art!'

'Please, Sir, instruct me further,' said Svetaketu.

'I shall, son,' Uddalaka replied.   (VI, xi, 3)

'Fetch me a fruit from that banyan tree.'

'Here it is, Sir.'

'Break it, son.'

'It is broken, Sir.'

'What do you see there?'

'Small seeds, Sir.'

'Break one of them.'

'It is broken, Sir.'

'What do you see there?'

'Nothing, Sir.'   (VI, xii, 1)

Uddalaka said : 'Son, from that subtle essence which you do not perceive there, from that very essence arises the great banyan tree. Believe what I tell you, son.'   (VI, xii, 2)

'In that which is the subtle essence, in that all that exists has its self. That is Truth. That is Self. That thou art!'

'Please, Sir, instruct me further,' said Svetaketu.

'I shall, son,' Uddalaka replied.   (VI, xii, 3)

'Put this salt in water; then see me in the morning,' Uddalaka said. Svetaketu followed his father's instruction.

In the morning, Uddalaka said : 'Please bring me the salt you put in the water last night.'

Svetaketu looked for the salt, but he could not find it, as it had completely dissolved.   (VI, xiii, 1)

'Take a sip from this end,' Uddalaka said. 'How does it taste?'

'It is salty,' Svetaketu said.

'Take a sip from the middle, and tell me how it tastes,' Uddalaka said.

'It is salty.'

'Now take a sip from the other end,' Uddalaka bade his son. 'How does it taste?'

'It is salty.'

'Throw the water away,' Uddalaka said, 'and come to me.'

Svetaketu did so, realizing : 'The salt continues to exist.'

Then Uddalaka said : 'My son, you do not perceive that Being here in this body, but verily, It is there.' (VI, xiii, 2)

'In that which is the subtle essence, in that all that exists has its self. That is Truth. That is Self. That thou art !'

'Please, Sir, instruct me further,' said Svetaketu.

'I shall, son,' Uddalaka replied. (VI, xiii, 3)

'As someone might lead a blindfolded person away from the province of Gandhara, and leave him in a deserted place; and as that person would turn round and round, shouting : "I have been brought here blindfolded! I have been left here blind-folded !" ' (VI, xiv, 1)

'And as thereupon someone might take off his blindfold, and tell him : "Gandhara is in that direction; go in that direction"; and as thereupon, if a sensible person, he would, by asking his way from village to village, finally arrive back in Gandhara – in exactly the same manner does a man who has found a teacher obtain true knowledge. For him there is delay only as long as he is not released from ignorance; after that he attains perfection.' (VI, xiv, 2)

'In that which is the subtle essence, in that all that exists has its self. That is Truth. That is Self. That thou art !'

'Please, Sir, instruct me further,' said Svetaketu.

'I shall, son,' Uddalaka replied. (VI, xiv, 3)

'Relatives gather round a dying person, asking : "Do you know me? Do you know me?" As long as his speech is not merged in his mind, his mind in *prana, prana* in fire, and fire in the highest deity, so long he knows them.' (VI, xv, 1)

'But when his speech is merged in his mind, mind in *prana, prana* in fire, and fire in the highest deity, then he does not know them any longer.' (VI, xv, 2)

'In that which is the subtle essence, in that all that exists has its self. That is Truth. That is Self. That thou art !'

'Please, Sir, instruct me further,' said Svetaketu.

'I shall, son,' Uddalaka replied. (VI, xv, 3)

'Son, they bring in an arrested man, saying : "This man has stolen something; he has committed a theft. Heat the hatchet for him."

If the man has committed the offence and denies it, then he is a
liar. Being given to falsehood, covering himself with a lie, he
grasps the heated hatchet – and is burnt. Then he is killed.'
(VI, xvi, 1)

'But if he did not commit the offence, then he is truthful. Being
given to truthfulness, clothing himself with truth, he grasps the
heated hatchet – he is not burnt, and he is freed.'　　(VI, xvi, 2)

'As the man who was not burnt lived in truth, so in that Being all
that exists has its self. That is Truth. That is Self. That thou art,
Sveta ketu!'

Then Svetaketu understood what was said; yes, he understood it.
(VI, xvi, 3)

Narada had approached the sage Sanatkumara, asking for instruction. These are the teachings of the sage on the Infinite:

'The Infinite is bliss. There is no bliss in anything finite. We must
desire to understand the Infinite.'

'Venerable Sir,' Narada said, 'I desire to understand the Infinite.'
(VII, xxiii)

'Where one sees nothing else, hears nothing else, knows nothing
else – that is the Infinite. Where one sees something else, hears
something else, knows something else – that is the finite. The
Infinite is immortal; the finite is mortal.'

'Venerable Sir, in what does the Infinite rest?' Narada asked.

'It rests in Its own greatness, and not even in greatness.'
(VII, xxiv, 1)

'In this world they call greatness the possession of cows, horses,
elephants, gold, slaves, wives, fields, or houses. I do not mean
greatness by this,' the sage spoke. 'For in these cases one thing
depends on another.'　　　　　　　　　　　　　　　(VII, xxiv, 2)

'The Infinite is below, above, behind, in front, on the right, on
the left. The Infinite is indeed all this.'

'Now follows the instruction of the Infinite as "I": I am below,
above, behind, in front, on the right, on the left. I am indeed all
this.'　　　　　　　　　　　　　　　　　　　　　(VII, xxv, 1)

'Next the instruction of the Infinite as the Self: The Self is below,
above, behind, in front, on the right, on the left. The Self is indeed
all this.'

'He who sees, feels, and knows this, he loves the Self, delights in
the Self, rejoices in the Self, revels in the Self. He becomes
independent; he moves at his pleasure in all the worlds.'

'But those who think differently from this are ruled by others. They live in perishable worlds, and they have no freedom.' (VII, xxv, 2)

'For him who sees, feels, and knows this, *prana* springs from the Self, hope springs from the Self, memory springs from the Self; ether, fire, water, appearance, disappearance, food, power, understanding, meditation, thought, will, mind, speech, names, sacred hymns, sacrifices – verily, everything springs from the Self.'

(VII, xxvi, 1)

'He who knows this, does not see death, nor disease, nor pain; he who knows this, knows everything, and obtains everything everywhere.' 'He is one, becomes three, becomes five, becomes seven, becomes nine; then he is called the eleventh, then the hundred and tenth, and the one thousand and twentieth.'

'When the intellectual food is pure, the mind becomes pure. When the mind is pure, memory becomes firm. When the memory remains firm, all ties are loosened.'

The venerable Sanatkumara showed Narada, after washing away his impurities, the other side of darkness. They call Sanatkumara *Skanda* [wise man]; yes, they call him *Skanda*.   (VII, xxvi, 2)

Prajapati spoke : 'The Self which is free from sin, old age, death, and grief, free from hunger and thirst, with true desires and true thoughts, that Self we must search for, that Self we must try to know. He who has searched for that Self and knows that Self, he obtains all worlds and all his desires.'   (VIII, vii, 1)

Both the gods and the demons heard these words, and they said : 'Let us search for this Self by the discovery of which all worlds are obtained, and all one's desires are fulfilled.'

Indra, king of the gods, and Virochana, king of the demons, both went, without having communicated with each other, to Prajapati, offerings in hand.   (VIII, vii, 2)

After they had remained for thirty-two years, practising continence, Prajapati asked : 'Why did you both stay here?'

They replied : 'You have said "The Self which is free from sin, old age, death, and grief, free from hunger and thirst, with true desires and true thoughts, that Self we must search for, that Self we must try to know. He who has searched for that Self and knows that Self obtains all worlds and all his desires." We have both stayed here because we desire that Self.'   (VIII, vii, 3)

Prajapati said : 'The person seen in the eye is the Self.' He added : 'He is the immortal, fearless *Brahman*.'

They asked : 'Venerable Sir, he who is seen in the water, and he who is seen in a mirror, who is he?'
Prajapati replied : 'He Himself is seen in all these.'   (VIII, vii, 4)

'Look at yourselves in a bowl of water. Whatever you then still do not understand about the Self, come and tell me.'
They looked at themselves in a bowl of water. Prajapati asked them : 'What do you see?'
They both replied : 'Venerable Sir, we see the complete self, a picture detailed to the very hairs and nails.'   (VIII, viii, 1)

Prajapati said : 'After adorning yourselves, after putting on your best clothes, and cleaning yourselves, look again into the water.'
After adorning themselves, after putting on their best clothes and cleaning themselves, they looked again into the bowl of water.
'What do you see?' Prajapati asked.   (VIII, viii, 2)

They replied : 'Just as we are adorned, dressed in our best clothes, and clean, Venerable Sir, thus we are both there, adorned, dressed in our best clothes, and clean.'
Prajapati said : 'That is the Self; that is the immortal, fearless *Brahman.*'
They both went away with satisfied heart.   (VIII, viii, 3)

Prajapati, seeing them go, said to himself : 'They both leave without having found, and without having known, the Self. Whoever follows their teaching, be he god or demon, will perish.'
Virochana, with satisfied heart, went to the demons, and taught them that the body alone is to be worshipped, that the body alone is to be served. He preached that he who worships and serves the body, gains both worlds, this and the next.   (VIII, viii, 4)

Hence even today they call a man who does not give alms, who has no faith, and who offers no sacrifices, a demon; for thus is the doctrine of the demons. They deck the bodies of the dead with perfumes, flowers, and fine raiment, thinking that they will conquer the next world.   (VIII, viii, 5)

But Indra, before reaching the gods, saw this difficulty : 'As this self, this reflection in the water, is well adorned when the body is well adorned, well dressed when the body is well dressed, clean when the body is clean, so this self will be blind if the body is blind, lame if the body is lame, crippled if the body is crippled, and will in fact perish when the body perishes. I cannot see any good in this doctrine.'   (VIII, ix, 1)

He returned with offerings in hand. Prajapati said to him : 'Indra, you left with Virochana, perfectly satisfied. Why did you come back?' Indra said : 'Venerable Sir, as this self, this reflection in the water, is well adorned when the body is well adorned, well dressed when the body is well dressed, clean when the body is clean, so this self will be blind if the body is blind, lame if the body is lame, crippled if the body is crippled, and will in fact perish when the body perishes. I cannot see any good in this doctrine.' (VIII, ix, 2)

'You are right, Indra,' Prajapati replied. 'I shall further explain the Self to you. Stay with me for another thirty-two years.' Indra stayed with Prajapati for another thirty-two years; then Prajapati said : (VIII, ix, 3)

'He who happily moves about in dreams, he is the Self; he is the immortal, fearless *Brahman*.'

Indra went away with satisfied heart. But before reaching the gods, he saw this difficulty : 'Though it is true that this self in dreams is not blind, not even when the body is blind, nor lame when the body is lame; though he does not suffer the defects of the body, (VIII, x, 1)

'nor is he struck when the body is struck, nor lamed when the body is lamed; yet it is as if they struck him, is as if they chased him. He becomes even conscious of pain, and sheds tears. I cannot see any good in this doctrine.' (VIII, x, 2)

He returned again with offerings in hand. Prajapati said to him : 'Indra, you left, perfectly satisfied. Why did you come back?' Indra said : 'Venerable Sir, though it is true that this self in dreams is not blind, not even when the body is blind, nor lame when the body is lame; though he does not suffer the defects of the body, (VIII, x, 3)

'nor is he struck when the body is struck, nor lamed when the body is lamed; yet it is as if they struck him, as if they chased him. He becomes even conscious of pain, and sheds tears. I cannot see any good in this doctrine.'

'You are right, Indra,' Prajapati replied. 'I shall further explain the Self to you. Stay with me for another thirty-two years.' Indra stayed with Prajapati for another thirty-two years; then Prajapati said : (VIII, x, 4)

'When a man is asleep, reposed, serene, and has no dreams, that is the Self; that is the immortal, fearless *Brahman*.'

Indra went away with satisfied heart. But before reaching the gods, he saw this difficulty : 'In fact, this self does not know himself as I, nor does he know anything at all. He has gone to utter annihilation. I cannot see any good in this doctrine.' (VIII, xi, 1)

He returned with offerings in hand. Prajapati said to him : 'Indra, you left, perfectly satisfied. Why did you come back?'
Indra said : 'Venerable Sir, in fact this self does not know himself as I, nor does he know anything at all. He has gone to utter annihilation. I cannot see any good in this doctrine.' (VIII, xi, 2)

'You are right, Indra,' Prajapati replied. 'I shall further explain the Self to you, and that will be the final explanation. Stay with me for another five years.'
Indra stayed with Prajapati for another five years. This made in all one hundred and one years; therefore people say that Indra stayed one hundred and one years as a celibate disciple with Prajapati. When the five years had passed, Prajapati said : (VIII, xi, 3)

'Indra, this mortal body is always under sentence of death, yet it is the abode of that deathless, bodiless Self. When the body is identified as the Self, the Self is thought to experience pleasure and pain. As long as He is thought to be the body, there are pleasure and pain. But when He is known to be independent of the body, then it is realized that neither pleasure nor pain can touch Him.'
(VIII, xii, 1)

'Wind has no body; clouds, lightning, and thunder have no bodies. Now, as these arise from yonder space and, on reaching their points of manifestation, appear in their own forms, (VIII, xii, 2)

'even so does that serene Being arise in this body when knowledge comes to its highest point, and appears in His own form. He is the supreme Soul. In that highest state He moves about, laughing, playing, rejoicing – be it with women, chariots, or relatives – heedless of that body into which He was born. As a horse is attached to the cart, so the *prana* animates this body.' (VIII, xii, 3)

'The gods in the world of *Brahma* meditate on that Self. Therefore they obtain all worlds and all their desires. He who knows and understands that Self obtains all worlds and all his desires.'
Thus spoke Prajapati; yes, thus spoke Prajapati. (VIII, xii, 6)

BRIHADARANYAKA UPANISHAD

There were two branches of descendants of Prajapati, namely the gods and the demons. The gods were the younger, and the demons he elder ones. They fought with each other for the possession of these worlds. The gods said : 'Let us overpower the demons at he sacrifice by means of the *Udgitha* chant.' (I, iii, 1)

They said to speech : 'Sing the *Udgitha* for us.'
Yes,' said speech, and sang the *Udgitha*. Whatever delight there is n speech, it secured for the gods by singing; that it spoke well, hat was for itself.
The demons knew that through this singer the gods would over->ower them. They rushed at the singer and pierced it with evil. Therefore the evil which consists in speaking what is bad, that is vil. (I, iii, 2)

Then the gods said to smell : 'Sing the *Udgitha* for us.'
Yes,' said smell, and sang the *Udgitha*. Whatever delight there is n smelling, it secured for the gods by singing; that it smelled well, hat was for itself.
The demons knew that through this singer the gods would over->ower them. They rushed at the singer and pierced it with evil. Therefore the evil which consists in smelling what is bad, that is vil. (I, iii, 3)

Then the gods said to sight : 'Sing the *Udgitha* for us.'
Yes,' said sight, and sang the *Udgitha*. Whatever delight there is n sight, it secured for the gods by singing; that it saw well, that vas for itself.
The demons knew that through this singer the gods would over->ower them. They rushed at the singer and pierced it with evil. Therefore the evil which consists in seeing what is bad, that is vil. (I, iii, 4)

Then the gods said to hearing : 'Sing the *Udgitha* for us.'
Yes,' said hearing, and sang the *Udgitha*. Whatever delight there s in hearing, it secured for the gods by singing; that it heard well, hat was for itself.
The demons knew that through this singer the gods would over->ower them. They rushed at the singer and pierced it with evil. Therefore the evil which consists in hearing what is bad, that is vil. (I, iii, 5)

Then the gods said to thought : 'Sing the *Udgitha* for us.'
Yes,' said thought, and sang the *Udgitha*. Whatever delight there s in thinking, it secured for the gods by singing; that it thought vell, that was for itself.
The demons knew that through this singer the gods would over->ower them. They rushed at the singer and pierced it with evil.

F

Therefore the evil which consists in thinking what is bad, that i
evil.
The demons touched all the other deities with evil, pierced ther
with evil. (I, iii, 6

Then the gods said to the vital breath: 'Sing the *Udgitha* for us
'Yes,' said the vital breath, and sang the *Udgitha*.
The demons knew that through this singer the gods would over
power them. They rushed at the singer to pierce it with evil. Bu
as a clod of earth is scattered when thrown against a rock, thu
the demons were scattered in all directions.
Therefore the gods triumphed, and the demons were destroyec
He who knows this triumphs in the Self, and the enemy wh
obstructs him is crushed. (I, iii, 7

While the priest chants, let the sacrificer recite these elevatin
mantras:

> Lead me from the unreal to the real!
> Lead me from darkness to light!
> Lead me from death to immortality!

When he recites: 'Lead me from the unreal to the real,' the unrea
verily means death, and the real, immortality. Therefore he :
saying: 'Lead me from death to immortality, make me immortal
When he recites: 'Lead me from darkness to light,' the darkne:
verily means death, and the light, immortality. Therefore he :
saying: 'Lead me from death to immortality.'
When he recites: 'Lead me from death to immortality,' no explana
tion is needed. (I, iii, 28

In the beginning, all this was Self alone, in the shape of a Persor
He looked and saw nothing but Himself. He first said: 'This is I
hence His name became I. Therefore even today if a man is aske
who he is, he first says: 'It is I,' and then gives whatever othe
name he may have. Because He destroyed all evil, He is calle
Purusha. He who knows this, destroys all evil. (I, iv, 1

He was afraid, and therefore people are afraid when alone. H
thought: 'Since there is only Me, of what am I afraid?' Thereupo
His fear passed away; of what should He be afraid? Verily, it is fo
a second only that fear arises. (I, iv, 2

He felt no happiness, and therefore a man is not happy when he i
alone. He desired a companion. He became as large as man an
wife in close embrace. He caused Himself to fall into two part
and thus husband and wife were born. Therefore, as the sag

Yajnavalkya has said, this body is one half of ourselves, like one of the halves of a split pea. Therefore the place of the other half is filled by the wife. He united with her, and man was born. (I, iv, 3)

She thought : 'How can He unite with me after producing me from Himself? I shall hide.'
She then became a cow; He became a bull, united with her, and cows were born. She became a mare, He became a stallion; she became a she-ass, He became a he-ass, united with her, and one-hoofed animals were born. She became a she-goat, He a he-goat; she became a ewe, He became a ram, united with her, and goats and sheep were born. Thus He created everything that exists in pairs, down to the ants. (I, iv, 4)

He knew that He was the creation, for He created all this. Therefore He became the creation, and he who knows this lives in this creation of His. (I, iv, 5)

Then by rubbing He produced fire from its source : the mouth and the hands. Therefore the mouth and the hands are hairless on the inside, for the inside of the fire-hole is without hair.
When they say : 'Sacrifice to this god,' or 'Sacrifice to that god,' these gods are but His manifestations; He is all these gods. (I, iv, 6)

This world was undifferentiated. It became differentiated by name and form; one could then say : 'He has such a name, such a shape.' Even to the present time everything is differentiated, and one can say : 'He has such a name, such a shape.'
The Self entered everything, to the tips of the nails. He lies hidden in everything, as a razor lies in its case, or fire in its source. People do not see Him, only in parts : when breathing He is called *prana,* the vital breath; when speaking, He is called speech; when seeing, light; when hearing, the ear; when thinking, mind. All these are but the names of His functions. He who regards Him as the one or the other does not know Him, for he regards only part of Him. Let men meditate on the Self, for in the Self all these are one – the Self is the footprint of everything, for through It one knows everything. As one can find again by its footprints that which was lost, thus he who knows this Self finds glory and freedom. (I, iv, 7)

This Self is dearer than a Son, dearer than wealth, dearer than everything else, and is innermost. If one said to a person who holds something other than the Self dear that he will lose what is dear to him, of a certainty he will lose it. Let him meditate on the Self alone as dear. He who meditates on the Self alone as dear, of a certainty what he holds dear will never perish. (I, iv, 8)

In the beginning this was *Brahman*. It knew Itself as 'I ar *Brahman*.' Everything sprang from this knowledge. Thus whateve god awakened to this knowledge, he became *Brahman*; it is th same with seers and men. Sage Vamadeva understood and sang 'I was *Manu* [moon], I was sun.' Also today he who thus realize that he is *Brahman*, becomes *Brahman*, and even the gods cannc prevent this, for he is also their Self.   (I, iv, 1(

As threads come forth from the spider, as small sparks come fort from the fire, so from this Self come forth all senses, all world all gods, all beings. Its name is 'Truth of truths.' The senses are th truth, and their truth is the Self.   (II, i, 2(

The description of *Brahman* is : 'Not this, not this,' for that is th highest description.
The name for *Brahman* is : 'Truth of truths,' the senses being th truth, and He being the truth of the senses.   (II, iii, (

The threefold offspring of Prajapati were gods, men, and demon They dwelt with Prajapati as celibate students. When they ha completed their terms, the gods said to Prajapati : 'Tell us, Sir Prajapati told them the syllable *da*, and asked whether they undei stood.
They replied : 'Yes, you told us *damyata* – control yourselves.'
Prajapati said : 'Yes, you have understood.'   (V, ii,

Then the men said to him : 'Tell us, Sir.'
To them he spoke the same syllable *da*, and asked whether the understood.
They replied : 'Yes, you told us *datta* – give.'
Prajapati said : 'Yes, you have understood.'   (V, ii, ;

Then the demons said to him : 'Tell us, Sir.'
To them he also spoke the syllable *da*, and asked whether the understood.
They replied : 'Yes, you told us *dayadhvam* – be compassionate.'
Prajapati said : 'Yes, you have understood.'
The heavenly voice of thunder repeats this same instruction '*D* da, da,' which means 'Control yourselves, give, be compassionate Therefore one should practise this triad of self-control, generosit and compassion.   (V, ii,

KAIVALYA UPANISHAD

Asvalayana asked the Lord Brahma : 'Venerable Sir, teach me th knowledge of *Brahman*, that knowledge which is supreme ar

hidden, constantly sought by the wise, that knowledge by which
the knower is freed from impurities and by which he attains the
greater than great Being.'   (1)

Brahma the grandsire spoke to him : 'Seek *Brahman* by faith,
devotion, meditation, and concentration. It is not obtained by
work, nor by offspring, nor by wealth; only by renunciation does
man achieve immortality.'   (2)

It is higher than heaven, shines in the lotus of the heart. Those
who struggle and aspire enter into It.'   (3)

In a solitary place, seat yourself in an easy posture, with pure
heart, with head, neck, and body straight, indifferent to the world,
controlling all the senses. Bow with devotion to the teacher.'   (5)

Devoid of passion and pure, meditate on the lotus of the heart,
in the centre of which is the pure, the sorrowless, the inconceivable,
the tranquil, the blissful, the source of Brahma.'   (6)

He is Brahma; He is Shiva; He is Indra; He is the Supreme; He
is Vishnu; He is *prana*; He is time; He is fire; He is the moon. (8)

He is all that has been, and all that will be. He is everlasting. By
knowing Him one conquers death. There is no other way to liberation.'   (9)

By seeing the Self in all beings, and all beings in the Self, one
goes to *Brahman*. There is no other way.'   (10)

Making the mind a firestick, and making the syllable *Om* a firestick; rubbing the two sticks together, by this effort kindling the
flame of knowledge, the knower burns all bonds.'   (11)

From Him are born life, mind, and the senses, earth, air, water,
fire, and ether. He is the support of all existence.'   (15)

He is the supreme *Brahman,* the Self of all, the foundation of all,
subtler than the subtle, eternal. That thou art, thou art That!' (16)

PAINGALA UPANISHAD

One should meditate upon these sacred sentences of the *Vedas* :

Tat tvam asi –	That thou art
Tvam tad asi –	Thou art That
Tvam brahmasi –	Thou art *Brahman*
Aham brahmasmi –	I am *Brahman*

The word *Tat* [That] denotes the cause of the universe, varied
beyond comprehension, having the qualities of omniscience, having
maya as vehicle, and having the attributes *Sat* [Being], *Chit*
[Consciousness] and *Ananda* [Bliss]. It is That which is the basis of
the I conception, and it is That which is denoted by the word
tvam [thou]. Undifferentiated *Brahman* remains after *maya* [illusory
principle] and *avidya* [spiritual ignorance], which envelop the
Universal Soul and the individual soul, respectively, are removed.

The investigation into the real meaning of the sentences *Tat tvam
asi* and *Aham brahmasmi* is what is called *shravana* [hearing].

Brooding on the meaning of what is heard is called *manana*
[reflection].

Concentrating the mind with one-pointedness on what is learned
through *shravana* and *manana* is *nididhyasana* [contemplation].

Samadhi is the state where there is no distinction between the
meditator and the act of meditation, and the mind resembles a lamp
in a windless spot. In that state arise the characteristics of the Self.
These characteristics cannot be known; they can be inferred only
from memory of the *samadhi* state. The innumerable *karmas* [net
works of results from past deeds] accumulated during this begin
ningless cycle of rebirth are destroyed through them. Through
efficiency in practice, a flow of nectar always rains down from
thousand directions. Therefore the yogis call this highest state
dharma-megha [cloud of virtue]. Through the manifestation of the
characteristics of the Self, the *karmas* are annihilated, leaving no
trace. When the good and bad *karmas* are totally destroyed, the
sentences *Tat tvam asi* and *Aham brahmasmi,* like objects in the
palm of the hand, give the yogi direct perception of *Brahman*,
though hitherto imperceptible. Then he becomes a *jivanmukti* [
liberated soul].   (III, 2

Being of pure mind, with purified consciousness, resigned, and
knowing 'I am He,' he should concentrate his heart on the Self.
Then he attains quiescence of the body, and mind and intellec
become still. Of what avail is milk to him who is filled with nectar?
Of what avail are the *Vedas* to him who knows the Self? For the
yogi who is filled with the nectar of the Knowledge of *Brahman*
there is nothing more to be achieved. If there is something still to
be achieved, then he is not a knower of *Tattva* [Truth]. Aloof, yet
not aloof, in the body, yet not restricted to the body, he is all
pervading. Having purified the heart and contemplated *Brahman*

the recognition of 'I' as the Supreme and the All is the highest
bliss. (IV, 9)

As water poured into water, milk into milk, *ghee* into *ghee,* so the
individual self and the Universal Self become one without differen-
tiation. (IV, 10)

Should a man perform *tapas* [austerity] standing on one leg for a
thousand years, this *tapas* will be worth not even a sixteenth of the
value of meditation. (IV, 15)

One who is desirous of knowing what constitutes *jnana* [spiritual
wisdom] and *jneya* [that which is to be known], will not attain his
desired end through the mere study of the *shastras* [scriptures], even
if he did so for a thousand years. (IV, 16)

That which *is* should be known as the imperishable. What appears
as the world is impermanent. Therefore, giving up the study of the
shastras, one should meditate upon Truth. (IV, 17)

Ceremonies, observances of purity, *japas* [repetitions of sacred sen-
tences], performances of sacrifice, and pilgrimages are all prescribed
as long as the seeker does not know Truth. (IV, 18)

For the great-souled, the realization 'I am *Brahman*' brings liberation. The sense of 'mine' leads to bondage, and the sense of 'not
mine' leads to liberation. (IV, 19)

Through the sense of 'mine' one is bound, and through the
absence of the sense of 'mine' one is liberated. When the mind
attains the state of enlightenment, the conception of duality is left
behind. (IV, 20)

When the seeker attains the state of enlightenment, he has attained
the highest state. Wherever his mind dwells, it dwells in the highest
state. (IV, 21)

That which is the same in all is *Brahman* alone. One may have
the power to strike the air with one's fist; one may be able to
appease one's hunger with the shells of grain, but one will never
attain emancipation if one has not the realization 'I am *Brahman*.'
(IV, 22)

CHAPTER ELEVEN

The Bhagavad Gita

The *Mahabharata* is a great epic which deals with the early history of India. It tells of the country's emperors, her brave warriors, her legends, her many sages, and her sublime spiritual teachings. Authorship of the classic is traditionally attributed to the legendary sage Vyasa, while the dates assigned to the work vary from 500 B.C. to as late as 200 B.C. The *Mahabharata* consists of about one hundred thousand couplets. The *Bhagavad Gita* forms a section of the sixth book of the epic.

Among the sacred books of the Hindus, the *Bhagavad Gita* occupies an honoured place. Great has been its influence throughout the ages, right up to the present time. To the venerated Mahatma Gandhi, the *Bhagavad Gita* was a never-ending source of inspiration. This man, so small in size and yet so great in stature, read from his beloved book every day. The appeal of the *Gita*, however is not specifically Indian, for its teachings are of universal interest, bound neither by age nor place. It has been called one of the world's greatest philosophical poems, and millions upon millions have found solace and inspiration from its pages.

Bhagavad Gita means 'The Lord's Song'. Extending to eighteen chapters, the book relates a discourse on the ways of action, devotion, and wisdom by the Lord Krishna to his disciple, the Prince Arjuna. The latter is a man at the psychological cross roads. He is about to do battle against many of his relatives. So far he has been a great warrior, fighting with bravery and skill, but suddenly the thought of having to engage in a fratricidal struggle becomes abhorrent to him. 'What good can come of killing one's relatives?' he asks. Overwhelmed by doubt and grief, he refuses to fight. Krishna consoles him. Arjuna is a soldier and, as he has right on his side, he must do battle. 'Stand up and fight!' Krishna urges.

At this point the spiritual teachings begin, and they occupy the rest of the poem. Some people, who undoubtedly meant well but probably never read further than the beginning of the second chapter, have expressed the opinion that the *Bhagavad Gita* is a book that urges us to fight and kill one another. That certainly is not the message of the *Gita* – on the contrary. The fact that in the first chapter the despondency of Arjuna is described with such feeling should be sufficient indication of the character of the book. The *Gita* has been lifted bodily from the *Mahabharata,* an epic; and the war merely provides the background for conveying spiritual teachings of the highest order. Arjuna happens to be a *kshatriya* – a member of the warrior caste – and as a soldier he must do his duty, just as each of us must perform his duty in the world. The real battle to be fought is against selfish desires, passion, and ignorance. Instead of hate, the *Gita* teaches all-embracing love.

The Yoga student will find much of great interest to him in the *Bhagavad Gita.* The book deals with Karma Yoga (the Yoga of Right Action) for those engaged in worldly activities; with Bhakti Yoga (the Yoga of Devotion) for those who are religious; and with Jnana Yoga (the Yoga of Knowledge) for those striving for spiritual wisdom.

The teachings of the *Gita* are based mainly on the *Upanihads,* and fundamentally the *Gita* teaches the transcendental *Brahman* of the *Upanishads.* 'The Upanishads are the cow, Krishna is the divine milker, the wise man is the drinker, and the nectarlike *Gita* is the excellent milk.'

It has been suggested that the *Bhagavad Gita* has not come down to us in its original form. During the passage of time, alterations are thought to have been made to the text, and the work perhaps was re-written several times in order to bring out specific views. This would partly account for the varying religious and philosophical expositions one finds side by side in the classic.

Following are excerpts from the *Bhagavad Gita.* Emphasis

in selection is on the teachings that fit most directly within the context of the present book.

THE BHAGAVAD GITA

On the field of righteousness, the plain of Kurukshetra, two opposing armies are drawn up, ready for battle. The struggle which is about to take place is the result of a long-standing feud between the Kurus and the Pandavas, members of two different branches of the same family. The Pandavas, to which the Prince Arjuna belongs, are fighting for the principle of righteousness Arjuna and his four brothers were brought up, together with their cousins, at the court of the father of these cousins, the King Dhritarashtra. Instead of giving up the throne as he should, being old and blind, Dhritarashtra wants to remain in power. Through continually favouring his own sons, the old King causes more trouble. After prolonged strife, the Pandavas are tricked and defeated by the Kurus at a dice game, whereupon, they are sent into exile. For more than twelve long years they wander, till at last war breaks out.

In order to make sure that the principle of righteousness prevails, Krishna, an *avatara* (divine incarnation) of Vishnu (one of the gods of Hinduism), manifests himself. An offer is made to both parties in the conflict. They may choose either a strong, well-equipped army or just himself, Krishna, a charioteer. The Kurus decide for the force of men and weapons while the Pandavas prefer to have the unarmed Krishna on their side.

Now the *Bhagavad Gita* begins. The opening verses tell of the many mighty warriors present, and describe battle preparations. The tumultuous sound of trumpets shakes the earth and the sky. In a great chariot, yoked with white horses, stand together the Lord Krishna and the Prince Arjuna:

Taking up his bow, Arjuna spoke to the Lord Krishna: 'Lord of the Earth! Please draw up my chariot between the two armies, O Changeless One,　　　　　　　　　　　　　　　　　　　(I, 21)

'So that I may look at those standing there, eager for battle, with whom I must compete in this outbreak of war;　　　　　　(I, 22)

"And gaze on those assembled, ready to fight and eager to please the evil-minded son of Dhritarashtra in the coming battle.' (I. 23)

Thus requested by Arjuna, the Lord Krishna drew up their bright chariot between the two armies.   (I, 24)

In front of Bhisma, Drona, and all the chieftains He spoke : 'Behold, O Arjuna, these Kurus assembled there.'   (I, 25)

Arjuna saw standing there fathers and grandfathers, teachers, uncles, brothers, sons and grandsons, friends;   (I, 26)

also in both armies were fathers-in-law and benefactors. Seeing all those kinsmen standing arrayed,   (I, 27)

Arjuna's heart melted with pity, and sadly he spoke : 'O Lord Krishna! When I see my own relations, ready and waiting for battle,   (I, 28)

'my limbs fail and my throat is parched; my body trembles and my hair stands on end;   (I, 29)

'the bow Gandiva slips from my hand, and my skin burns all over. I cannot stand up, and my mind is reeling.'   (I, 30)

'I see adverse omens, O Krishna! Neither do I foresee any good from slaying my own people in this fight.'   (I, 31)

'O Lord! I desire neither victory, nor kingdom; nor do I crave for pleasure. What is a kingdom to us, O Krishna, or enjoyment, or even life?'   (I, 32)

'Those for whose sake we desire kingdom, enjoyment, and pleasure, they stand here ready for battle, prepared to abandon life and riches—   (I, 33)

'teachers, fathers, sons, and grandfathers, uncles and fathers-in-law, grandsons, brothers-in-law, and other relatives.'   (I, 34)

'Though they might kill me, I do not wish to kill them, O Krishna, not even for the kingdom of the three worlds – how much less than for this earth?'   (I, 35)

'What happiness can be ours, O Lord, when we slay these sons of Dhritarashtra? We shall sin if we kill these people.'   (I, 36)

'Therefore we should not kill these sons of Dhritarashtra, our kinsmen; for how can we obtain happiness, O Lord, from the destruction of our relatives?'   (I, 37)

'Although these men, blinded by greed as they are, see no wrong in the destruction of a family, and no crime in hostility to friends,
(I, 38)

'we, who see evil in the destruction of a family – should not we turn away from so great a sin?'   (I, 39)

'Verily, it would be far better for me if the sons of Dhritarashtra, weapons in hand, should slay me in battle, unarmed and un-resisting.'   (I, 46)

Having thus spoken, on the field of battle, Arjuna, casting away bow and arrow, sank on the seat of the chariot, overwhelmed by sorrow.   (I, 47)

To him who was thus overcome by pity, whose eyes were dimmed with tears, and who was so despondent, the Lord Krishna spoke these words :   (II, 1)

'O Arjuna! Whence comes in this critical hour this dejection, which is unworthy of Aryans, and which leads only to disgrace and closes the gates of heaven?'   (II, 2)

'Yield not to weakness, O Arjuna! It does not befit thee. Rid thy-self of this despicable faint-heartedness and arise, O conqueror of foes!'   (II, 3)

Arjuna replied : 'O Lord! How can I attack Bhisma and Drona with arrows in battle – those who are worthy of reverence, O Destroyer of the enemy?'   (II, 4)

"Better were it to eat a beggar's crust in this world than to slay these honoured teachers; if I killed these instructors of mine, life's pleasure would be stained with blood.'   (II, 5)

'Nor do I know which is the better for us – that we conquer them or that they conquer us. We should not care to live if we slayed these sons of Dhritarashtra, albeit they stand arrayed against us'   (II, 6)

'My heart feels faint, and my mind is confused as to what my duty is. I implore Thee, O Lord, which is the better for certain, for I am Thy disciple. I have take refuge in Thee; please teach me.'   (II, 7)

'For I see not what would remove this anguish which withers my senses, even should I attain unrivalled and prosperous mastery on earth, or even mastery over the gods.'   (II, 8)

Having thus addressed the Lord Krishna, the conqueror of foes said : 'I will not fight,' and became silent.   (II, 9)

Thereupon, between the two armies, the Lord Krishna, with understanding smile, spoke to him who was so despondent. (II, 10)

'Thou grievest for those for whom thou shouldst not grieve, and yet thou speakest of wisdom. The wise grieve neither for the dead nor for the living.'   (II, 11)

'Never was there a time when I was not, nor thou, nor these princes; never will there be a time when we shall cease to be.'
(II, 12)

'Contacts of the senses with their objects bring cold and heat, pleasure and pain. They come and go, and do not last forever. Endure them bravely, O Prince !'   (II, 14)

'He who is not afflicted by these, who remains balanced in pleasure and in pain, only he is fit for immortality.'   (II, 15)

'That which is not, shall never be; that which is, shall never cease to be. To the seer, these truths are apparent.'   (II, 16)

'That, which pervades all this, is immutable. Nothing can destroy That.'   (II, 17)

'The bodies, in which the Eternal, Indestructible and Incomprehensible dwells, are all finite. Therefore fight, O Prince !' (II, 18)

'He who regards That as slaying, and who regards That as slain, they are both ignorant. That slayeth not, nor is It slain.' (II, 19)

'That was not born, nor does It die; nor having been will That ever cease to be; unborn, eternal, perpetual, and primeval, That is not slain when the body is destroyed.'   (II, 20)

'He who knows That as indestructible, perpetual, unborn, and unchanging, how could he kill, O Prince, or cause to be killed?'
(II, 21)

'Just as a man casts off worn-out garments, and puts on others which are new, so That throws off worn-out bodies, and enters into others which are new.'   (II, 22)

'Weapons cleave That not, fire burns That not; water cannot wet That, and wind cannot dry That.'   (II, 23)

'That is uncleavable, cannot be scorched, nor wetted, nor dried. That is eternal, all pervading, unchanging, and immovable.'
(II, 24)

'That is called the Unmanifest, the Unimaginable, and the Immutable. Therefore, knowing That as such, thou shouldst not grieve.'
(II, 25)

'Even if thou thinkest of That perpetually being born and perpetually dying, even then, O Prince, thou shouldst still not grieve.'
(II, 26)

'For death is certain for that which is born, and certain is birth for that which is dead. Therefore grievest not for the inevitable.'
(Il, 27)

'Beings are unmanifest in their beginnings, manifest in their interim states, O Prince, and unmanifest again in dissolution. What cause is there then for grief?'
(II, 28)

'Some regard That as marvellous; others similarly speak of That as marvellous; as marvellous some hear of That; yet after having heard, few indeed understand That.'
(II, 29)

'The Dweller in the body of everyone, O Prince, is ever invulnerable. Therefore thou shouldst not grieve for any creature.'
(II, 30)

'Thou must look at thy duty, and thou shouldst not waver, for nothing could be more welcome to a brave soldier than a righteous war.'
(II, 31)

'Fortunate indeed are the soldiers, O Prince, to whom such an unsought fight offers the opportunity to enter the open gate of heaven.'
(II, 32)

'Shouldst thou not take part in this righteous war, then thou forsakest thy duty and thy honour, and thou shalt incur only sin.'
(II, 33)

'Men will forever speak of thy dishonour; and to the highly-esteemed, dishonour is worse than death.'
(II, 34)

'The great charioteers will think thou hast fled from battle through fear; though once thought of highly, thou wilt then be but lightly esteemed.'
(II, 35)

'Thy enemies will speak ill of thee, slandering thy strength. What could be more humiliating?'
(II, 36)

'If killed in battle, thou shalt obtain heaven; if victorious, thou shalt enjoy the earth. Therefore, O Prince, stand up and fight.'

(II, 37)

'Looking equally upon pleasure and pain, gain and loss, victory and defeat, gird thee for battle, for thou shalt incur no sin.'   (II, 38)

'Thus I have told thee the wisdom of Samkhya. Now hear the teaching of Yoga, through the application of which, O Prince, thou shalt cast away all bonds of action.'   (II, 39)

'On this path, no effort is ever lost, nor is there transgression. Even a little of this righteousness delivers one from the great fear.'

(II, 40)

'The resolute mind, O Prince, is but one-pointed; the thoughts of the irresolute wander into bypaths innumerable.'   (II, 41)

'Fools utter flowery speech, O Arjuna, and are satisfied with the mere letter of the *Vedas,* saying that there is nothing but this.'

(II, 42)

'Full of selfish desires, intent on a temporary heaven, they offer rebirth as a result of action, and prescribe arduous and complex rites for the attainment of pleasure and power.'   (II, 43)

'Their minds clinging to enjoyment and power, and captivated by such, they cannot engage in concentration leading to *samadhi.*'

(II, 44)

'Rise above the three Vedic qualities of nature, O Arjuna! Be above the dualities; steadfast in purity, be free of desires for material possessions, and centred in the Self.'   (II, 45)

'To the *brahmana,* the knower of Truth, all the *Vedas* are of as little use as is a well to one who stands surrounded by water.'

(II, 46)

'Thou hast right only to action, and never to its fruits. Let therefore not the fruit of action be thy motive; neither be thou attached to inaction.'   (II, 47)

'Fixed in Yoga, do thy work, O Prince! Abandoning attachment, be balanced equally in success and failure. Even-mindedness is called Yoga.'   (II, 48)

'Action is far inferior to the Yoga of Intelligence, O Arjuna! Have recourse then to pure intelligence. Pitiable are they who seek the fruit of action.'   (II, 49)

'Having attained Knowledge, one abandons in this world both good and evil. Therefore engage thyself in this Yoga. Skill in action is called Yoga.'   (II, 50)

'The wise, having attained Knowledge, renounce the fruits of action. Freed from the bonds of birth, they reach the highest bliss.'   (II, 51)

'When thy intellect escapes the tangle of delusion, then thou shalt become indifferent to expositions heard and yet to be heard.'   (II, 52)

'When thy mind, at first confused by the various texts of the scriptures, stands immovably in *samadhi,* then thou hast attained Yoga.'   (II, 53)

Arjuna asked : 'How do we know him who is steadfast of mind and who has attained *samadhi,* O Lord? How does he speak, how does he sit, how does he walk?'   (II, 54)

The Lord Krishna replied : 'When a man has given up all desires, O Prince, and is content only in the Self, then he is called steadfast of mind.'   (II, 55)

'He whose mind remains unruffled in pain, and whose desire for pleasure has been overcome, he in whom passion, fear, and anger have been subdued, he is called a sage of steadfast mind.'   (II, 56)

'He who is free from all attachment, who neither rejoices on receiving good nor hates on receiving bad, his wisdom is established.'   (II, 57)

'He who withdraws his senses from the surrounding objects of sense as the tortoise draws its limbs within its shell, his wisdom is established.'   (II, 58)

'Objects of sense, if not the desire for them, turn away from him who is austere of habit. Even the desire for objects of sense is killed after the Supreme is seen.'   (II, 59)

'The tumultuous senses, O Prince, impetuously carry away the the mind, even of the discriminating man striving for perfection.'   (II, 60)

'Having brought all the senses under control, he should sit firm, meditating on Me, the Supreme Goal; for he whose senses are mastered, his wisdom is established.'   (II, 61)

'Musing on objects of sense, man becomes attached to them. From attachment arises desire, and from desire springs anger.'   (II, 62)

'From anger comes delusion, delusion results in confused memory, confused memory shatters reason, and with the shattering of reason man perishes.'   (II, 63)

'But the disciplined soul, moving amongst objects of sense with senses under control and free from attraction and aversion, attains eternal peace.'   (II, 64)

'In that peace there is extinction of all misery, and the peaceful mind soon becomes established in wisdom.'   (II, 65)

'There exists no reason for the uncontrolled, nor is there meditation for the uncontrolled. Without meditation there is no peace, and without peace, how can there be happiness?'   (II, 66)

'As a boat on the waters is blown along by the wind, so reason is carried away from the mind that yields to the roving senses.'

(II, 67)

"Therefore, O mighty-armed, he whose senses are detached from the objects of sense, his wisdom is established.'   (II, 68)

'What is obscure to the unenlightened is clear to the disciplined soul; and what is real to the world is illusion to the *muni* [sage] who sees.'   (II, 69)

'He attains peace who remains unaffected by desires, as the ocean, filled with water, remains ever the same though rivers flow into it; but not he who maintains desires.'   (II, 70)

'He who gives up desires, and goes his way free from desires, selfishness and egotism, he attains peace.'   (II, 71)

'This is the state of *Brahman*, O Prince! Having attained it, one is never again confused. When one becomes established in this state, if even at one's last moments, one attains *brahmanirvana* [beatitude of *Brahman*].'   (II, 72)

Arjuna queried : 'If Thou considerest knowledge superior to action, O Lord, why then dost Thou instruct me to engage in this terrible fight?'   (III, 1)

'With seemingly contradicting words Thou confusest my reason; therefore please tell me decisively by which way I may attain the highest.'   (III, 2)

The Blessed Lord replied : 'As I declared, in this world there is a twofold path, O sinless one. There is Jnana Yoga for the contemplative, and Karma Yoga for men of action.'   (III, 3)

'A man cannot achieve freedom from action merely by refraining from action, nor does he rise to perfection by mere renunciation.'   (III, 4)

'Nor can anyone remain actionless, not even for a moment; for all are compelled to act by the qualities of nature.'   (III, 5)

'He who sits with organs of action controlled, but with his mind dwelling on objects of sense, that confused soul is simply called a hypocrite.'   (III, 6)

'But he whose mind has command of the senses, O Arjuna, and who detachedly engages the organs of action in Karma Yoga, such a man excels.'   (III, 7)

'Perform thou *karma* [right action], for right action is superior to nonaction; even the body cannot be maintained if one refrains from action.'   (III, 8)

'In this world one is bound by one's actions, unless such actions are performed in a spirit of sacrifice. Therefore, O Prince, perform thy actions without attachment.'   (III, 9)

'He who rejoices only in the Self, who is satisfied and content with the Self alone, for him nothing remains to be done.'   (III, 17)

'He need not concern himself with action nor with nonaction in this world; nor does he depend on any creature.'   (III, 18)

'Therefore always, without being attached, perform the work that has to be done, for by detachedly performing action, man attains the Supreme.'   (III, 19)

'King Janaka and other great souls attained perfection through right action alone. Even for the benefit of the world thou shouldst perform right action.'   (III, 20)

'Whatever a great man does, that others do. Whatever standard he sets is followed by the world.'   (III, 21)

'There is nothing in the three worlds, O Prince, that I need do nor is there anything to be attained which has not yet been attained; yet I still engage in action.'   (III, 22)

'For should I not engage in action untiringly, O Prince, men everywhere would follow my example.' (III, 23)

'Should I cease to act, these words would be destroyed through confusion, and I should be the author of the destruction of these people.' (III, 24)

'As the ignorant act because of atachment to action, O Prince, so the wise should act without such attachment, desiring only the welfare of the world.' (III, 25)

'The man of wisdom should not perturb the minds of the ignorant who are attached to action; instead he should act in harmony, and cause others to be desirous of engaging in right action.' (III, 26)

'All actions are the products of the *gunas* [qualities of nature], but the soul deluded by egotism thinks "I am the doer".' (III, 27)

'He, O mighty-armed, who knows correctly the relationship between the *gunas* and action, realizing that the *gunas* act according to their respective character, he is not attached.' (III, 28)

'Those deluded by the *gunas* are attached to the actions of the *gunas*. However, let not the man who knows unsettle the minds of those who know little.' (III, 29)

'Offering all thy actions to Me, with mind fixed in the Self, not thinking of reward, free from egotism, and delivered from grief, engage thou in battle.' (III, 30)

Arjuna asked : 'By what is a man driven to sin, O Krishna, as if compelled, and even against his wishes?' (III, 36)

The Blessed Lord replied : It is lust, it is hate, springing from the *rajas guna* [quality of darkness]; all-consuming, all-corrupting, know this as thy foe here.' (III, 37)

'As fire is shrouded by smoke, as a mirror is covered by dust, and as an embryo is enveloped in the womb, so the world is wrapped in desire.' (III, 38)

'Desire envelops wisdom, and is the constant enemy of the wise, O Arjuna! Desire is as insatiable as fire.' (III, 39)

'The senses, the mind, and the intellect are said to be its seats; veiling wisdom by these, it deludes man.' (III, 40)

'Therefore, O Prince, first control thy senses, and then slay this sinful destroyer of *jnana* [spiritual knowledge], and *vijnana* [scientific knowledge].'   (III, 41)

'It is said that the senses are powerful, but superior to the senses is the mind; the intellect is superior to the mind, but greater than the intellect is the Supreme.'   (III, 42)

'Thus knowing the Supreme to be greater than the intellect, and subduing the personal ego by the Self, slay desire, O mighty-armed, this enemy so hard to overcome.'   (III, 43)

'What is action, and what is inaction? This question has confounded even the wise. I shall tell thee what is action, and knowing thou shalt be delivered from evil.'   (IV, 16)

'It is essential to know what constitutes right action, and what wrong action. Likewise one should know what is inaction, for mysterious is the path of action.'   (IV, 17)

'He who sees inaction in action, and action in inaction, he is wise among men. He is balanced in all his actions.'   (IV, 18)

'Him whose actions are all undertaken free from the motive of desire, whose actions are burned by the fire of wisdom, him the sages call wise.'   (IV, 19)

'Having abandoned attachment to the fruits of action, ever content and independent, though he acts he acts not.'   (IV, 20)

'Expecting nothing, controlled and steady, having abandoned all greed, thus performing bodily action only, he remains untainted.'
     (IV, 21)

'Content with whatever may happen to come to him, risen above the dualities, free from envy, equal-minded in success and in failure, he is not bound by his actions.'   (IV, 22)

'He who has overcome attachment, who is liberated and whose mind is established in wisdom, who acts in a spirit of sacrifice, his actions leave no binding consequences.'   (IV, 23)

'For him, *Brahman* is the act of offering as well as the oblation. *Brahman* is both the sacrificer and the sacrificial fire. He shall go to *Brahman* who during all his actions meditates upon *Brahman*.'
     (IV, 24)

'Some yogis offer sacrifices to the *devas* [gods]; others sacrifice by the act of sacrificing in the fire of the Supreme.'   (IV, 25)

'Some offer, as sacrifice, hearing and the other senses in the fire of self-control; others offer, as sacrifice, sound and the other objects of sense in the fire of the senses.'   (IV, 26)

'Others again offer all the functions of the senses and of the life-force in the wisdom-kindled fire of the Yoga of self-control.'
(IV, 27)

'There are those who offer as sacrifice wealth, austerity, or medita-tion; while others, restrained and holding to severe vows, offer their study and learning as sacrifice.   (IV, 28)

'Some pour as sacrifice *apana* [the outgoing breath] into *prana* [here : the incoming breath] and *prana* into *apana*. Thus having restrained the flow of both *prana* and *apana,* they are entirely absorbed in *pranayama.*'   (IV, 29)

'Others, curbing their intake of food, offer as sacrifice their life-breath into life-breaths. All these know sacrifice, and by sacrifice they destroy their sins.'   (IV, 30)

'Drinking the nectar of the remains of the sacrifice, they attain *Brahman.* This world is not for him who offers no sacrifice; how much less then is any other world, O Prince?'   (IV, 31)

'Thus many forms of sacrifice are set forth as the means of attain-ing *Brahman.* Know that all these are born of action, and knowing thus thou shalt be free.'   (IV, 32)

'Greater than any material sacrifice is the sacrifice of spiritual wis-dom, O Arjuna, for the whole realm of action culminates in that wisdom.'   (IV, 33)

'Learn thou this by obeisance, by inquiry, and by service. The wise, having realized Truth, will instruct thee in *jnana* [spiritual know-ledge].'   (IV, 34)

'Knowing it, thou shalt not again fall into delusion, O Prince, for by that wisdom thou shalt see all creatures without exception in the Self – that is in Me.'   (IV, 35)

'Be thou of all sinners the most sinful, thou shalt cross over the ocean of sin by the raft of *jnana.*'   (IV, 36)

'As the kindled fire burns the fuel to ashes, O Arjuna, so does the fire of *jnana* reduce all actions to ashes.'   (IV, 37)

'Nothing in this world is so purifying as *jnana;* and he who is perfected by Yoga finds it in due time in the Self.'   (IV, 38)

'He who is of unflinching faith, and who has control over his senses, he obtains *jnana*. Having obtained *jnana,* he swiftly goes to eternal Peace.'   (IV, 39)

'The ignorant, the faithless, and the doubters will perish. For him who doubts, there is neither this world nor beyond, nor is there any happiness.'   (IV, 40)

'He who has renounced actions by Yoga, who has cut asunder doubt by *jnana,* and who always has his mind fixed in the Self, he is not bound by actions, O Prince!'   (IV, 41)

'Therefore, cleaving asunder with the sword of *jnana* this doubt in the heart, which is born of ignorance, practice Yoga and arise, O Prince!'   (IV, 42)

Arjuna said : 'O Krishna! Thou praisest both the renunciation of actions and Yoga. Please tell me conclusively which the better of the two.'   (V, 1)

The Blessed Lord replied : 'Renunciation and Karma Yoga [the selfless performance of right action] both lead to the highest bliss. Of these two, verily Karma Yoga is superior to renunciation of action.'   (V, 2)

'Know him as a *sannyasi* [a true renouncer] who neither hates nor desires; not influenced by dualities, O Prince, he is easily freed from bondage.'   (V, 3)

'It is the ignorant, and not the wise, who speak of *Samkhya* [here : the intellectual approach to renunciation] and Yoga [here : Karma Yoga] as different. He who establishes himself in one, obtains the fruits of both.'   (V, 4)

'The height obtained by *samkhyas* [see previous verse] is also achieved by yogis [see previous verse]. He who sees that Samkhya and Yoga are one, he sees.   (V, 5)

'But indeed, O mighty-armed, renunciation is hard to achieve without the practice of Yoga. The *muni* [sage], firmly established in Yoga, swiftly attains *Brahman.*'   (V, 6)

'He who is established in Yoga, who is purified, who has subdued personal ego and senses, who knows his soul to be the Self of all beings, even though acting, he is not affected.'   (V, 7)

' "I do not anything," the yogi, knower of Truth, should think, though seeing, hearing, touching, smelling, eating, moving, sleeping, and breathing.' (V, 8)

'Though speaking, emitting, grasping, opening and closing the eyes, he maintains that it is merely the senses that are occupying themselves with the objects of sense.' (V, 9)

'He who acts, non-attached, dedicating all his actions to *Brahman*, he is unaffected by sin, as the leaf of the lotus remains dry in the water.' (V, 10)

'Karma yogis, abandoning all attachment, perform action with the body, the mind, the intellect, and the senses only, and always as a means of purification.' (V. 11)

'The yogi, having abandoned the fruit of action, attains eternal peace; he who is not a yogi is impelled by desire and, attached to the fruit of action, he is bound.' (V, 12)

'Having mentally renounced all action, the self-controlled embodied one resides serenely in the city with the nine gates (the physical body with its nine apertures), neither acting nor causing action.' (V, 13)

'Neither action nor cause of action flows from the Supreme Self, nor does the relationship between action and its fruit emanate from the Supreme Self; it is nature which manifests all these.' (V, 14)

'The all-pervading Self partakes not of anyone's sin, nor even of his virtue. Wisdom is covered by ignorance, and subsequently men are deluded.' (V, 15)

'Verily, for those in whom ignorance has been destroyed by *jnana*, for those *jnana* reveals the highest.' (V, 16)

'Meditating on That, and believing only in That, established in That and holding That as their supreme goal, they attain a state from which there is no return, their sins dispelled by *jnana*.' (V, 17)

'Sages look equally upon a learned and humble *brahmana* [knower of *Brahman*], a cow, an elephant, or even a dog or an outcaste.' (V, 18)

'Earthly existence is overcome even while here on earth by those whose minds are established in equality. *Brahman* is equal and without blemish; therefore they are established in *Brahman*.' (V, 19)

'The steady-minded and unperplexed knower of *Brahman*, being established in *Brahman*, neither rejoices on receiving the pleasant nor sorrows on receiving the unpleasant.'   (V, 20)

'He who is unattached to external contacts and who finds joy in the Self, whose self is united with *Brahman* through Yoga, he enjoys imperishable bliss.'   (V, 21)

'The pleasures that spring from external contacts are only sources of unhappiness, for they have their beginnings and their endings, O Arjuna; the wise do not rejoice in them.'   (V, 22)

'He who is able to withstand the forces of desire and anger, even here on earth before he leaves the body, he is a yogi, and a happy man.'   (V, 23)

'He who is happy within, who finds joy within, and whose light shines within, that yogi attains *brahmanirvana* [beatitude of *Brahman*] and he becomes *Brahman*.'   (V, 24)

'*Rishis* [seers], with sins washed away and dualities destroyed, who are controlled, and who take pleasure in the welfare of all beings, they attain *brahmanirvana*.'   (V, 25)

'*Brahmanirvana* is near for the ascetics who have control over their minds, who have overcome desire and anger, and who have knowledge of the Self.'   (V, 26)

'Excluding the outside world, with gaze fixed between the eyebrows, the incoming and outgoing breaths flowing evenly through the nostrils, with senses, mind, and intellect controlled, the goal liberation, the *muni* [sage], having cast away desire, fear, and anger, is forever free.'   (V, 27, 28)

The Blessed Lord spoke : 'He who performs actions because they are his duty, and not for the fruits of such actions, he is a *sannyasi* and a yogi; not so he who does not burn the sacrificial fire and who is without action.'   (VI, 1)

'What they call renunciation, know thou that as Yoga, O Prince, for no one can become a yogi who has not given up all selfish purposes.'   (VI, 2)

'For the meditator who seeks to attain Yoga, practice is called the means; when he has attained Yoga, serenity is the sign.'   (VI, 3)

'When a man is no longer attached to objects of sense nor to actions, when he has renounced all selfish purposes, then he is said to have attained Yoga.'   (VI, 4)

'He who has conquered his personal ego, and who dwells peacefully in the Supreme Self, he is balanced in heat and cold, in pleasure and pain, in honour and dishonour.' (VI, 7)

'He who is satisfied with wisdom and spiritual knowledge, who is steadfast and master of his senses, to whom a clod of earth, a stone, and a piece of gold are the same, he is said to be joined in Yoga.' (VI, 8)

'He excels who looks equally upon lover, friend, and foe; upon strangers, neutrals, foreigners, and relatives; upon the virtuous as well as upon the sinner.' (VI, 9)

'Let the aspirant constantly concentrate his mind, seated in solitude in a secluded place, self-controlled, and free from desire and from longing for possessions.' (VI, 10)

'In a clean place, having established his own firm seat, not too high and not too low, with cloth, skin, and grass placed over one another, (VI, 11)

'seated there, having made his mind one-pointed, and with thought and senses subdued, let him practice meditation for self-purification.' (VI, 12)

'Let him hold body, head, and neck erect, remain motionless and look fixedly between the eyebrows with unseeing gaze.' (VI, 13)

'Calm and fearless, observing celibacy, with mind controlled, let him sit steadfastly, and meditate and aspire toward the Supreme.' (VI, 14)

'The yogi, thus ever balanced and controlled, attains the eternal peace that abides in the Supreme.' (VI, 15)

'Verily, Yoga is not for him who eats too much, nor for him who fasts to excess. It is not for him who sleeps too much, nor for him who keeps awake too long, O Arjuna!' (VI, 16)

'But for him who is moderate in food and pleasure, who is controlled in behaviour and action, who has regulated his sleeping and his waking, for him Yoga becomes the destroyer of all sorrow.' (VI, 17)

'When the subdued mind rests in the Self alone, free from all desires, then that sage is said to be joined to the Self.' (VI, 18)

'Steady as a lamp in a sheltered spot is the yogi of subdued thoughts who practices union with the Self.' (VI, 19)

'Where the mind comes to rest, curbed by practice; where he beholds the Self with his whole being, and rejoices in the Self;

(VI, 20)

'where he experiences an infinite bliss which transcends the senses and which can be grasped only by the *buddhi* [higher intelligence]; and from where, once established, he never again moves away from Truth;   (VI, 21)

'beyond which, having gained it, he thinks there is no greater gain; wherein established, he is disturbed not even by the greatest sorrow;   (VI, 22)

'let that stage be known as Yoga, this dissociation from pain. This Yoga should be practised with determination and cheerful mind.'

(VI, 23)

'Abandoning completely all desires born of selfishness, curbing with the mind all the senses in every way;   (VI, 24)

'little by little, let him attain tranquillity by means of reason controlled by steadiness; having made his mind meditate upon the Self, let him not think of anything else.'   (VI, 25)

'Wheresoever the wavering and unsteady mind runs, let him restrain it and bring it back from there to the meditation upon the Self.'   (VI, 26)

'Supreme bliss comes to the yogi whose mind is peaceful, whose passions have subsided, who is sinless, and who has become one with *Brahman*.'   (VI, 27)

'Thus, constantly in harmony, free from sin, the yogi easily enjoys the ultimate bliss that springs from contact with *Brahman*.'

(VI, 28)

'He who is harmonized by Yoga sees the Self abiding in all beings, and all beings in the Self; everywhere he sees oneness.'   (VI, 29)

'He who, knowing the same Self to dwell in everything, sees equality everywhere, O Arjuna, be it pleasurable or painful, he is considered a true yogi.'   (VI, 32)

Arjuna said : 'This Yoga, founded on even-mindedness, which has been declared by Thee, O Lord, I see not how it is possible, owing to restlessness.'   (VI, 33)

'For restless indeed is the mind, O Krishna; impetuous, strong, and obstinate, I deem it as hard to restrain as the wind.'   (VI, 34)

The Blessed Lord spoke : 'Doubtlessly, O mighty-armed, the restless mind is hard to restrain; but it may be controlled, O Arjuna, by constant practice and nonattachment.' (VI, 35)

'Yoga is difficult to attain by one who is not self-controlled; but for those who are self-controlled it is attainable through striving correctly.' (VI, 36)

The Blessed Lord spoke : 'I shall now declare that which is to be known, and by knowing which, immortality is enjoyed. It is beginningless and supreme *Brahman,* called neither being nor nonbeing.' (XIII, 12)

'With hands and feet everywhere, with eyes, heads, mouths, and ears everywhere, It dwells in the world, enveloping all.' (XIII, 13)

'Endowed with the faculties of the senses, yet without the senses, unattached yet sustaining everything, devoid of *gunas* [qualities of nature] yet the enjoyer of the *gunas;* (XIII, 14)

'beyond and inside all beings, moving and unmoving, too subtle for comprehension, near and far, is That.' (XIII, 15)

'Indivisible, yet present in separate beings, It is to be known as the Sustainer, the Destroyer, and the Creator.' (XIII, 16)

'Light of lights, beyond darkness, *jnana* [spiritual knowledge], object of *jnana,* and to be attained by *jnana,* That is seated in the hearts of all.' (XIII, 17)

'He who sees that it is *prakriti* [nature] that performs all actions, and that the Self is not acting, he truly sees.' (XIII, 29)

'When he sees the diversity of existence as being seated in One, and as sprouting forth from One, then he becomes *Brahman.*' (XIII, 30)

CHAPTER TWELVE

Integration

According to Sankaracharya, four qualifications are required of one who desires to know the nature of the Self. The renowned sage lists these four qualifications in his *Viveka Chudamani* (19-28).

1. *Viveka* – Discrimination.
   The student should learn to distinguish that which is permanent from that which is transient. He should know the Real from the unreal.

2. *Vairagya* – Nonattachment.
   Whether the student follows the path of *Raja Yoga* or that of *Jnana* Yoga, he must overcome all desire for, and attachment to, worldly objects. The paths of *Raja* and *Jnana* Yoga run parallel.

3. *Shatsampatti* – Six attributes, which are :
   shama – control over the mind and the ability to concentrate.
   dama – control over body and senses.
   uparati – self-reliance, the state of not being dependent on anything or anyone.
   titiksha – forbearance, the state of mind in which one can endure all pain and sorrow without malice, dejection, or lamentation.
   shraddha – faith in the masters' teachings as set out in the scriptures.

164

samadhana – the ability to hold the mind steady on the Self, with total disregard for things of a worldly nature.

4. *Mumukshutva* – Ardent desire for spiritual emancipation through knowledge of one's true self.

The student should devote some time each day to reading the scriptures, and to meditating on the meaning of what is read. The utterances of the sages on *Brahman* should become his sustenance.

With the true recognition of the nature of *Brahman,* all is known. The knower has become a yogi, having *Brahmavidya* (knowledge of *Brahman*). Nothing more remains to be known, and nothing more to be achieved. He has merged with Universal Life, as rivers, losing name and form, become one with the sea.

Dualities have dissolved into *Brahman.* Where others see differences and separateness, the yogi sees Oneness, knows Oneness, and feels only Oneness. His notion of individual existence has been destroyed; his personality expands into *Brahman.* The Yogi can truly say: *'Aham brahmasmi'* ('I am *Brahman*').

The yogi's life is an example of harmony. He acts in harmony with his surroundings, or harmoniously he refrains from action. 'As birds and deer avoid a burning mountain, so sins do not touch those who know *Brahman*' (*Maitri Upanishad,* VI, 18).

Although the yogi has transcended his limitations, he is a humble person. Others may wonder at his self-control and his self-reliance, yet he may speak little of his exalted state. How can others possibly understand the privileged condition in which he finds himself? It is all one to him whether he retires from the world, or whether he participates in worldly affairs. In the midst of all activities, his mind dwells upon the Eternal. He is in constant meditation, at all times abiding in *Brahman.* No matter what he does, or does not do, his mind is always anchored in the bliss of Existence. He is in this world, but not of it. Though outwardly acting as if with attachment, he is unattached at heart. The clothes which cover his physical body may vary with the country in which he lives, but internally he always wears the yellow robe.

The yogi has a deep love for humanity, as he has for all creatures. He feels his kinship with all life, expressed and unexpressed. He sees the One Life manifesting Itself in the multitude of transient modes of existence. The knower of *Brahman* experiences wholeness. He has become an integrated universal being, a true cosmic man.